ETHICS

PROFESSIONAL ISSUES

Also in this series

Nurses and Patients
Aspects of Nursing Care
Nursing People with Special Needs – Part I
Nursing People with Special Needs – Part II
Education and Research
Conflicts of Interest

ETHICS
PROFESSIONAL ISSUES

Edited by

Verena Tschudin BSc(Hons), RGN, RM, Dip. Counselling

Illustrations by Richard Smith

Scutari Press · London

© Scutari Press 1995

A division of Scutari Projects Ltd, the publishing company of the Royal College of Nursing.

All rights reserved. No part of this publication may be reproduced, stored in a retrieval system or transmitted in any form or by any means, electronic, mechanical, photocopying or otherwise, without the prior permission of Scutari Press, Viking House, 17/19 Peterborough Road, Harrow HA1 2AX, England.

First published 1995

British Library Cataloguing in Publication Data
Professional Issues. – (Ethics Series)
  I. Tschudin, Verena II. Smith, Richard
  III. Series
  174

ISBN 1-873853-14-9

Phototypeset by Intype, London
Printed and bound in Great Britain by
Athenaeum Press, Gateshead, Tyne and Wear

Contents

Contributors vi
Preface vii
1 **The Control of Professional Behaviour** 1
    Ann P Young
2 **Standards of Practice** 36
    Betty Kershaw
3 **Professionalism and Professional Qualifications** 61
    Betty Kershaw
4 **Independent Midwifery Practice** 84
    Caroline Flint
Index 115

Note: Page 88 line 3 for *syntometrine (hastening labour)* read *syntometrine (oxytocic)*.

Contributors

Ann P Young   BA, RGN, RNT

Senior Lecturer, East London Business School, University of East London

Betty Kershaw   RGN, RNT, MSc(Nursing)

Director of Nurse Education, Manchester College of Midwifery and Nursing

Caroline Flint   SRN, SCM, ADM

Independent Midwife, Honorary Professor, Thames Valley University

Preface

Ethics is not only at the heart of nursing, it *is* the heart of nursing. Ethics is about what is right and good. Nursing and caring are synonymous, and the way in which care is carried out is ethically decisive. How a patient is addressed, cared for and treated must be right not only by ordinary standards of care, but also by ethical principles.

These ethical principles have not always been addressed clearly, but now patients, nurses, doctors and all types of health care personnel are questioning their care in the light of ethics. Their starting points and approaches are different, but their 'results' are remarkably similar. The individual person matters and the care given and received has to be human and humanising.

The way in which the contributors to this volume, and others in the series, address their subject is also individual and unique. Their brief was simply that what they wrote should be applicable to practising nurses. Each chapter reflects the personal style and approach of the writer. This is what gives this series its distinctive character and strength, and provides the reader with the opportunity to see different approaches working. It is hoped that this will encourage readers to think that their own way of understanding ethics and behaving ethically is also acceptable and worthwhile. Theories and principles are important, and so are their interpretation and application. That is a job for everybody, not just the experts: experts can point the way — as in this series of books — but all nurses need to be challenged and encouraged.

Emphasis is laid in all the chapters on the individual nurse and patient or client. Ethics 'happens' between and among people, and, by the authors bringing their own experience to bear on their chapters, they show how ethics works in relationships.

Great achievements often start with a small idea quite different from the end result, and so it is with this series of books. The initial proposal is almost unrecognisable in the final product. Many people contributed to the growth of the idea, many more were involved in implementing it, and I hope that even more will benefit from it.

My particular thanks go to Geoff Hunt, Director of the European Centre for Professional Ethics, for his advice and help with this series.

Verena Tschudin

CHAPTER 1
The Control of Professional Behaviour
Ann P. Young

> Professional practitioners work within frameworks that they need both to keep and respect, and also interpret and question. These frameworks of codes and legislation are intended to shape and form a profession, and the author of this chapter appeals to these aspirations in her conclusions. Not only do authors and teachers have to recognise the ideal and the possible, but also every practitioner has a responsibility to enable better care and practice by being aware of legal and practical controls. Some of the practical controls of nursing lie in its culture of often punitive and prescriptive customs from a bygone age, which neither codes nor education have yet managed to sweep away. This chapter concentrates on the tangible controls of professional nursing practice, while not dismissing the intangible and often implicit controls.

How nurses give care is strongly influenced by the social, professional and personal frameworks within which they operate. This chapter will explore the methods that society uses to influence or control individual behaviour, how this applies to nursing, whether such frameworks hinder or enhance the quality of care given and whether they impinge in a positive or negative way on professional autonomy.

Methods of Social Control

From a very early age, a child is socialised into behaving in a way that is acceptable to its parents. Punishment and reward play a part in shaping how a child acts, as does following the example presented by the parent as a role model. This shaping continues as the child lives through school years, with informal pressures and formal rules. Initially, children may need to conform consciously to the social expectations surrounding them, but much behaviour is then internalised and no longer has to be consciously carried out. In adulthood, further socialisation takes place at work or through leisure activities.

Within a relatively cohesive society, such socialisation processes will be of major importance in maintaining order. However, it is a rare society that can rely totally on such methods, hence the development of formal rules drawn up, perhaps, for specific groups within society (eg certain religious groups) and on a national or international level. This development of control mechanisms can be traced in many countries. The extension and coordination of common rules or laws across England came about as travel and trade increased contacts between small communities, and the need for stability and peace within the evolving society of the 12th century was seen as important. The roots of much of today's English law were laid down at that time as common law and have continued to develop to the present day (Padfield 1983).

Although some rules governing behaviour are seemingly imposed on people, they often arise from basic ethical premises held by a large number of individuals within that society. For example, in England, causing damage to people or their belongings is seen almost as an absolute wrong that must be punished. It is possible to envisage a society that does not accept such a premise. A society which allows cannibalism or supports public ownership of all property would clearly be very different. Other ethical thinking that underlies some UK rules is the concept of fairness or equity and the promotion of the greatest good. The former is seen in much employment law, and the latter is seen as an influence on the distribution of scarce resources.

Some tentative conclusions can, therefore, be drawn from the discussion so far. Firstly, any society will exercise control on individual members in order to maintain stability and the existing power structure. Secondly, the nature of the controls will be mixed. Laws are the most rigid and can be applied relatively evenly across a nation and even more widely (though usually less successfully) across a number of states. Ethical norms are likely to exist, although it is unlikely that these will be accepted by all. The education process must be considered important in developing norms of behaviour, and the state may have some control through curriculum requirements. However, the most important context in which behaviour is learned and internalised is the family unit. External control is limited, with parental influence often a repeat of previously learned patterns of behaviour, whether useful or destructive.

The Nature of Professional Behaviour

Members of a profession undertake work of a particular nature, and professions are characterised by the provision of some kind of personal service that requires a high level of specialised knowledge and skill. As this puts professionals in a position of power over clients receiving the service, a profession will develop means of controlling its members in order to safeguard clients.

Characteristically, a profession only allows its practitioners full entry on completion of a set course of approved study and passing of examinations. Disciplinary measures will be taken against members who fail to abide by a code of conduct drawn up by the profession. Using these criteria, nursing is a good example of a profession.

However, it is something of an anomaly that these very

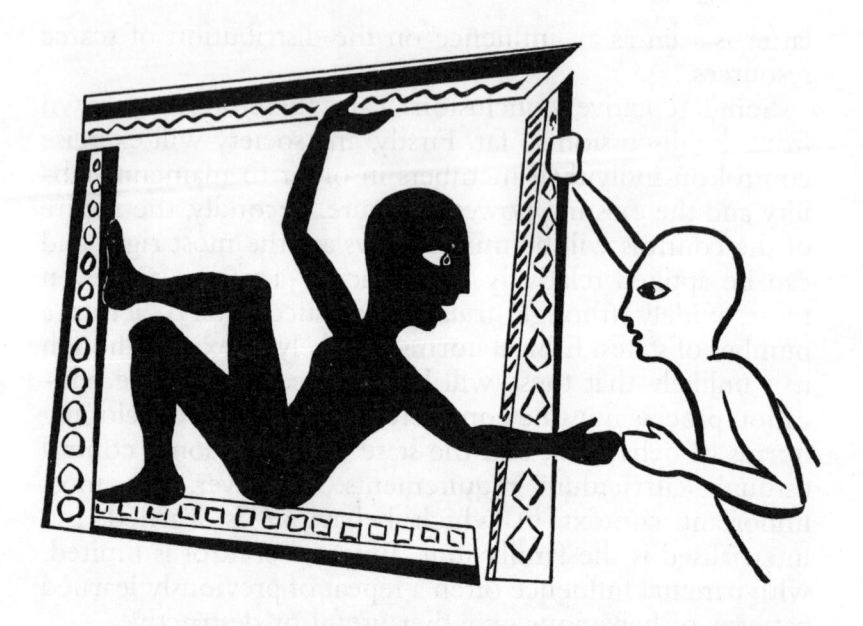

measures of exerting some control over the individual tend to promote a perception of self that values individuality and autonomy (Handy 1985). General managers in the NHS have found to their cost that whereas it is relatively simple to persuade administrative staff to abide by new procedures, professional staff (most notably doctors) resent externally imposed rules and are quite capable of sabotaging the best-laid plans if they feel that they have not been consulted and involved in the decision-making.

The nature of professional training and work, therefore, tends to reinforce the links and loyalties with other similar professionals rather than with the professional's own workplace, leading to the possibility of conflicting control mechanisms between profession and employer. It is likely that with the major changes now implemented in the NHS (National Health Service and Community Care Act 1990), the forces of the internal market may reinforce the importance of loyalty to the organisation in order to promote its survival (and therefore one's own continuing employment). Teamwork across professional and non-professional boundaries is becoming more widely accepted for the enhancement of patient care, and one possible outcome may be a reduction in the professional elitism and isolation from non-professionals currently in existence. Such changes will undoubtedly have an effect on control mechanisms.

Controls on Professional Behaviour

The influence and effectiveness of various social controls will now be explored in more depth, relating these specifically to nursing.

Legal Controls

As citizens nurses have to abide by the law of the land.

A basic classification divides law into criminal and civil law (Young 1989). A criminal offence is committed against the state and is punishable by the state. Nurses may become involved in this type of law in relation to drugs and theft. Civil law, on the other hand, involves the rights and duties of individuals towards each other. Legal action is taken by a private individual rather than the state, and the outcome of such an action would be the award of some monetary compensation. This type of law is particularly important to nurses since the area of negligence is a major influence on nurses' behaviour. There are areas of overlap between criminal and civil law. For example, assault and battery can be both a criminal and a civil wrong, and gross negligence may become a crime, such as manslaughter, if the patient dies.

Another way of classifying law is into statute and case

law. Whereas case law has its roots in the old common law and was largely unwritten, statute law is developed through parliament. The latter has become increasingly important as a source of law in this century, but, for the nursing and medical professions, case law as it is developed by judges through the court system is very influential in interpreting and clarifying much of the law relating to patient care.

A critical analysis of these legal controls is outlined below.

Statute law

There are a number of statutes that affect how nurses behave towards their patients or clients.

The Mental Health Act 1983 underpins much of the care given by nurses in the psychiatric area, and, in spite of recent criticisms, does much to both safeguard the public and enhance patients' rights. Getting the balance right is never going to be easy, but the pressure to alter the Act to include greater statutory controls has, rightly, been seen as inappropriate. The issue is more one of functioning without adequate resources, and changes to the law are not addressing the root cause of the problem.

The National Health Service and Community Care Act 1990 is one of the most far-reaching statutes affecting patient care since the original NHS Act of 1946. The division between purchasers and providers of care, and the transfer of some responsibilities for long-term care from the NHS to the social services sector, has changed the orientation within the NHS to a business and marketing environment. While this approach has the advantage of promoting efficiency, the speed of the changes has created many difficulties, not least the fear that quality issues are seen as less important than financial ones.

Other recent statutes of wide-ranging importance to nurses are the Access to Health Records Act 1990, the

Hospital Complaints Procedure Act 1985 and the Children Act 1989.

Professionals need to view legislation in two ways, considering, firstly, how to abide by the law and, secondly, how to influence the formation of new law through the parliamentary process.

The need to abide by the law seems almost too obvious. However, one of the difficulties that nurses encounter is that statute law is not always easy to read or interpret. Nurses, therefore, rely heavily on others to explain the implications of legislation. In addition, no statute can ever be fully comprehensive, and, therefore, ongoing interpretation is necessary in specific types of work or variable situations. It may be necessary for further legal clarification to take place through the court system, but often the development of codes and guidelines plugs the gaps.

Traditionally, nurses have been slow and ineffective in influencing the formation of new law. The largely female workforce, supported by a number of unions and professional bodies, has tended to lead to a passive approach without a clear voice (Salvage 1985).

However, statute law can be influenced in a number of ways. In each parliamentary session, a number of members of parliament are entitled to introduce a Private Members Bill. Much lobbying of these MPs occurs in order to interest them in particular issues. The success rate of Bills introduced in this way is not high, owing to the pressures on parliamentary time, but even those that fail may raise sufficient public and parliamentary awareness for them to be introduced as a Government Bill at some point. The amendments to the 1967 Abortion Act are a good example of this. The Alton Bill failed through purposeful time-wasting tactics by those opposed to it, with the government then taking it up and getting the changes through in the Human Fertilization and Embryology Act 1990.

Government-supported legislation usually starts with

the production of a White Paper. This is a detailed proposal that is published before the Bill itself is drafted and presented to parliament. Comments made at this stage may influence the exact format of the Bill. Other influence can be exerted by ensuring that the professional's own MP is aware of her or his views, which could affect some of the details within a Bill at committee stage. Obviously, it is more effective for nurses to form a pressure group than to act individually.

There is, therefore, the possibility of statute law being modified between its inception and the point at which it is enacted. Much detailed work takes place at the committee stage, out of sight of the general public, and the debates taking place in both the House of Commons and the House of Lords can be useful for thrashing out various points. However, the strengths of the UK legislative procedures are weakened by the time constraints in operation.

Case law

Case law is particularly important in influencing the care that patients receive.

The law on negligence relies heavily on case law, which has defined and applied this concept to patient care over the years. In *Blyth* v. *Birmingham Waterworks Co. Ltd.*, 1856, negligence was defined as 'the omission to do something which a reasonable man, guided upon those considerations which ordinarily regulate the conduct of human affairs, would do, or doing something which a prudent and reasonable man would not do' (Pannett 1992). Several further cases clarified that negligence consists of three elements: a duty of care, breach of that duty by act or omission, and resultant harm.

Lord Atkin in *Donaghue* v. *Stevenson*, 1932, defined the duty of care: 'the rule that you are to love your neighbour becomes in law that you must not injure your neighbour'. But who is my neighbour? The answer in law is, 'persons who are so directly affected by my act that I ought reasonably to have them in contemplation as being so affected when I am directing my mind to the acts or omissions which are called in question' (Pannett 1992).

As the concept of negligence became applied to patient care, a wealth of case law developed to set the standard of care expected from the professional person. Probably the most important case is *Bolam v. Friern Hospital Management Committee*, 1957. The judge stated that 'the medical standard of care is the standard of a reasonably skilled and experienced doctor', and 'it is well established law that it is sufficient if he exercises the ordinary skill of an ordinary competent man exercising that particular art' (Mason and McCall Smith 1987).

Case law has also played an important part in the development of the law relating to patient consent for adults, children and those who are suffering some mental incapacity. In addition, case law is also often used to clarify statute law.

The use of case law in influencing patient care has a number of advantages. It makes for flexibility in the interpretation of the law without having recourse to parliament and the long-winded route through legislation. It ensures that professionals can have a voice in influencing the law through the evidence that they give in court, not through evidence of facts, but of opinion. The use of expert witnesses to put forward what would be the accepted standard of care in various circumstances is well established.

However, there are limitations to the value of case law, particularly for the nursing profession. There are only a limited number of cases involving nurses that are heard in court, and, therefore, much of the law relating to patient care has been developed in relation to medical care. The conclusions reached must then be applied to the nursing context.

For case law to be developed, a case must also be heard in sufficiently high a level of court for the outcome to create a legal precedent, ie a conclusion that then becomes binding on similar cases heard in lower courts. When a particularly important issue has to be settled, the case may be purposely referred to the House of Lords (the highest court in the land) in order to create as binding a precedent as possible, which is what happened in *Airedale NHS Trust v. Bland*, 1993 (Dyer 1992).

The quality of the case law developed depends on the expert witnesses called, and this may not be done with impartiality where contentious issues are to be heard (as possibly in the Dr Arthur case in 1981, involving the death of a handicapped baby; Skegg 1984). It also depends on the judges hearing the case; they may not be without their own values and beliefs which colour the judgements that they make (Skegg 1984).

As with statute law, case law has to be understood and applied across a variety of situations. Additional guidelines are, therefore, often needed.

Delegated legislation

The drawback of legislation is the time taken either to get a Bill presented to parliament or, once presented, successfully to complete all the stages required for its acceptance.

A certain amount of law is, therefore, enacted through delegated legislation. For nurses, this is an extremely important route for legislation to take, as the Nurses Rules binding much of nursing's professional status are a form of delegated legislation through statutory instruments. The enabling Act is the Nurses, Midwives and Health Visitors Act 1979 (amended 1992).

The United Kingdom Central Council (UKCC) set up under this Act is empowered to draw up these Rules, which become law once approved by the Secretary of State. This body of 40 elected and 20 appointed members is a potentially powerful group of people affecting the nursing profession. The introduction of Project 2000 training was the result of prolonged consultation by the UKCC with members of the profession and other interested parties (UKCC 1986). A similar process is under way to amend post-registration education and practice (PREP, UKCC 1993).

The UKCC also has an important remit to protect the public from incompetent practitioners. As well as controlling training and registration, it performs this function through professional discipline. These issues are further discussed later in this chapter.

The statutory power given to the nursing profession to control its own affairs in this way is important, not only to nurses, but also to the patients they care for. However, criticisms have been made of the professional imbalance of the Council members elected in 1993, with the areas of mental health and learning difficulties very underrepresented. The percentage of registered nurses, midwives and health visitors voting at the last election was also disappointingly low. Seemingly, not all nurses value the potential for power and influence that they can exert in this way.

Overall, the Nurses, Midwives and Health Visitors Act gives the profession a wide statutory remit to regulate itself by 'establishing and improving standards of training and professional conduct' (Nurses, Midwives and Health Visitors Act 1979). Quite how it does this has changed over the years and will continue to change as the profession increasingly seeks and expects its statutory body to be both responsive and proactive through the major changes of the last decade of the 20th century.

The European Union

The Treaty of Rome was originally signed in 1957, bringing together six European countries. The UK joined in 1973, and British subjects have since then been increasingly influenced by European Union (EU) legislation. The Single European Act 1987 and ratification of the Maastricht Treaty in 1993 have strengthened the economic and legislative links between the UK and other member states of the EU.

There are a number of ways in which behaviour is controlled by Community legislation. Regulations are directly applicable in all member states and do not have to be confirmed by national parliaments in order to have a binding legal effect. If there is conflict between a regulation and an existing national law, the regulation prevails.

Directives produced by the Council of Europe are binding but require to be implemented through the member state's own legislative processes. This type of European law is particularly important in health care. A number of Directives on health and safety were brought into action in January 1993 through UK regulations. These are somewhat wider in scope than the Health and Safety at Work Act 1974 and have an important effect on how nurses work, for example in moving and handling patients (National Back Pain Association 1992).

EU decisions, recommendations and opinions can also influence local national law.

There has been some doubt as to the full implications of EU legislation on the UK, but the situation has been clarified through case law. For example, in employment law, a number of Directives have resulted in UK regulations that have been more restrictive than the original Directives. Case law has underlined the fact that if national regulations fail to implement fully the requirements of the Directive, it is the Directive that will then be binding in the UK (Dwan 1992).

To many, the development of law in this way seems rather distant and the European Parliament, Council and Commission, inaccessible. However, influence can be exerted through the UK parliament in a similar way. EU legislation is subject to scrutiny by parliament, and there is a select committee on European legislation for each House. Individuals are entitled to voice their views either to these committees, to their own member of parliament, or directly to Brussels.

Codes, Policies and Guidelines

There are many other controls on nurses' behaviour apart from those with legal power. Codes, policies and guidelines vary as to their impact, depending on the context in which they exist. A number of these are now discussed.

Professional codes

One of the hallmarks of a profession is that it has a code of conduct.

One of the earliest codes influencing nurses was that produced by the International Council of Nurses. The 1973 version (the most recent) covers five main areas: nurses and people, nurses and practice, nurses and society, nurses and co-workers and nurses and the profession (ICN 1973). This code provides *guidance* to nurses, and failure to follow it carries no penalty.

Much better known to UK nurses is the UKCC Code of Professional Conduct (1992a). Previous editions were 'issued for guidance', as one would expect of a code. However, the wording of the 1992 (3rd) edition has been subtly altered in that it 'requires members to practise and conduct themselves within the standards and framework provided by the Code'. Thus, the Code is, in fact, used as a standard against which to judge professional misconduct leading to the possible ultimate punishment of removal of a nurse's name from the Register.

This seems to lift the status of the Code to one that is not far off the force of legal rules, as removal from the Register is certainly a legal outcome, preventing the individual from practising. However, as with the law, the difficulty facing professionals is in interpreting the Code within the context of a wide variety of settings and circumstances. The UKCC has published a number of additional guidelines for standards, giving more detailed advice for interpreting the Code, for example, the interpretation of the nature of the nurse's accountability (UKCC 1989), advice on how to reach conclusions in relation to patient confidentiality (UKCC 1987) and some ground rules on how to deal with advertising and commercial sponsorship (UKCC 1990).

Some aspects of the Code have definite links with the law. Following the 'stem sentence' 'As a registered nurse, midwife or health visitor, you are personally accountable for your practice and, in the exercise of your professional accountability, must ...', Clause 2 states: 'ensure that no action or omission on your part, or within your sphere of responsibility, is detrimental to the interests, condition or safety of patients and clients'. This has marked similarity to the law of negligence, and, in fact, a number of other clauses are well supported by case law in this area. For example, the law requires the professional to keep up to date in practice, and the Code requires the nurse to 'maintain and improve professional knowledge and competence'; the law expects the standard of care to be that of the reasonably skilled qualified person, while the Code requires nurses to 'decline any duties or responsibilities unless able to perform them in a safe and skilled manner' (Young 1994).

However, some clauses repeatedly cause nurses difficulty. For example, 'report to an appropriate person or authority, having regard to the physical, psychological and social effects on patients and clients, any circumstances in the environment of care which could jeopardise standards of practice' (clause 11) and 'any circumstances in which safe and appropriate care for patients and clients cannot be provided' (clause 12) seem to be particularly prone to variable interpretations. The measurement of what constitutes safe care is probably the least contentious in the above, but nurses usually expect or hope to be able to achieve a higher standard than merely 'safe'. Interpretation of 'appropriate' will probably vary depending on whose perspective is taken — medical, managerial, the patient's or the practising nurse's, to name just four potentially differing views.

A possible way out of this dilemma is not to rely on one individual's interpretation but to use discussion and debate between a group of professionals to reach consensus on what may be seen as an acceptable and appropriate standard in different circumstances. Such a route would rely on openness in working relationships, whereas trust can be eroded when pressure rises to meet financial targets through staff cutbacks.

A further difficulty revolves around identifying who is the 'appropriate person or authority'. If the first step of reporting to one's immediate manager fails to result in any kind of reasonable response, the individual will then need to involve a higher level of management. Without support, nurses may fear later victimisation from following this route, although a failure to do so could put them in breach of the Code of Conduct. Again, the best advice is to take concerns to management in a group rather than alone, or at least with the support of a union or professional organisation.

Some employers are beginning to appreciate the important influence of the Code of Professional Conduct on its nursing workforce. A requirement to abide by the Code has been incorporated in some employment contracts, raising the status and force of the Code. However, these employers are in the minority, and conflicts between the contractual and professional position of nurses still occur.

Employment codes and policies

Statute law often needs further clarification, and this is sometimes done through case law. However, in the area of employment, further interpretation and guidance may take the form of codes of practice or local policies.

The Advisory, Conciliation and Arbitration Service (ACAS) has drawn up a number of codes of practice to give both employers and employees guidelines in interpreting legislation. Several codes relate to the Employment Protection (Consolidation) Act 1978 and, although not legally enforceable, will be used within an industrial tribunal or appeal setting to illustrate whether the employer followed good practice or not. An employer shown to have ignored codes of practice may not lose the case but will be criticised. This may make for bad publicity, and most organisations are conscious of the fact that to recruit and retain good staff, they need to promote a positive image.

Although codes of practice will, therefore, have some influence on the workplace, it is a fact that parts of the Employment Protection (Consolidation) Act 1978 have been interpreted through the courts in a way that often seems more supportive of employer authority than employee protection (Bowers 1990). This is particularly apparent in the area of unfair dismissal. The 'some other substantial reason' of Section 57(1)b has been widened to justify a dismissal as fair to include, for example, reorganisation of the workforce, a frequent occurrence these days!

For nurses, it is important to be able to feel some employment security, as the fear of termination of employment may otherwise impinge on how they can function professionally. The clause quoted in the previous section (reporting any circumstances jeopardising standards) is a good example here. Fear of unwanted employment consequences may lead to more acquiescence to authority than is in the patients' interests.

Union activity

Union activity can be valuable, not just in supporting individual members, but also in balancing the power between employees and employers and thereby giving employees a stronger voice within the organisation. Again, codes of practice are valuable here in giving guidelines as to when paid and unpaid leave should be given to shop stewards. (Dimond 1990). For example, it is suggested that stewards should be allowed paid leave for union activities directly related to employment. The time off should be 'reasonable', and the code puts responsibility on the manager to ensure that cover is provided in the nurse's absence.

Industrial action is an area where emotions run high. Strike action could be detrimental to patient care, and a code of practice supports professionals in not having to take action conflicting with the conduct laid down by their statutory body. If nurses still decide to take industrial action, the UKCC Code of Professional Conduct must be adhered to by not acting in a way that may be 'detrimental to the condition or safety of patients and clients' (clause 2).

Local rules and policies

An employee's behaviour will also be influenced by local rules. Most contracts of employment will make reference to disciplinary rules, with information as to where these may be found. This is in line with the Employment Protection (Consolidation) Act 1978 (Section 1.4). These rules are drawn up for several reasons. They assist in the promotion of fair treatment of employees, as well as ensuring that workers and managers can operate within an ordered framework. They are also an important way of ensuring that certain standards are met. Of relevance to nurses are those relating to health and safety and aspects of patient care such as confidentiality. Breach of these rules could lead to dismissal, and this will be clearly stated and be a part of the employee's contract of employment.

The process of drawing up local rules and policies will indicate how much influence individual employees have on the final outcome. The process is usually initiated by senior management who perceive a need for regulation in some area of work. Draft rules are prepared. Usually, some consultation of experts takes place at this point. For example, rules relating to discipline, sickness or union activity may be prepared by the human resource department, while rules controlling some aspect of patient care will be written with the advice of practitioners. The drafts then go through a process of consultation. Practice may vary considerably as to the extent of consultation. Union leaders, managers and other specifically involved groups should be enabled to comment, but the rights of employees (except through their union membership) may be limited.

Comments received will be considered and may be incorporated into the final version. The rule or policy will then be officially approved at executive level and information relayed to all employees. If the comments received raise some serious issues about the draft, it may need to be amended and go out for a further consultative period before being finally accepted. As can be seen, the process of producing local rules or policies can be long-winded, although the incorporation of the right to consultation maintains the possibility of some employee influence.

With the NHS facing so much rapid change, there is a temptation to shortcut the processes described above in order to produce quick regulatory mechanisms. Senior management may respond to a crisis situation by looking to amend a policy when other action may be more appropriate. For example, there has been wide publicity of some NHS Trusts introducing 'gagging' clauses into employees' contracts, making the divulging of confidential material outside the organisation a serious offence likely to lead to dismissal. However, nurses have always been bound to confidentiality by their Code of Conduct. Perhaps it would be more appropriate for management to examine its internal mechanisms for dealing with staff complaints about standards of care and promoting a more open climate of debate within the organisation, rather than reacting defensively to criticism.

However, the time scale taken to produce local policies can be a valid criticism of management. The current trend of producing standards of performance as part of a quality assurance programme moves away from rules controlling many facets of employee behaviour to broad policies providing principles on which to base local decisions. Again, the introduction of a quality approach involving all members of staff is time-consuming, but in the long run it is more likely to be effective and, just as importantly, flexible and responsive to changing circumstances.

Once local rules and policies have been introduced, the issue is one of enforcing them. As already explained, these local rules are contractually binding, although the issue is rarely that simple. Conformity by employees will tend to occur only if the rule is seen to be sensible and understandable. Many organisations are littered with rules that are regularly flouted and about which little is done. For example, uniform regulations are frequently ignored. Nurses fail to realise the health and safety implications of local rules, many of which are unfortunately lengthy and based on tradition and emotion rather than common sense. To single out one individual for discipline tends to lead to the cry of 'but everybody does/doesn't do this', and although such an argument can never be an acceptable reason for not punishing misconduct, the manager would be wise to consider quite what the 'misconduct' is and why it has occurred.

Making the 'punishment fit the crime' is also important. Employee perceptions of misconduct may differ from those of management, for example on the acceptable level of sickness. Guidelines setting likely standards are important, but a very rigid interpretation of these may lead to unfairness.

In conclusion, local rules and policies must be seen to apply to areas of importance, be relevant and clearly understandable. Processes including employee consultation and involvement are more likely to lead to the production of sound rules than is the imposition of decisions made by senior management alone. Employee cooperation and conformity are then more likely to follow.

Guidelines for practice

At intervals, various bodies issue guidelines that have an influence on the work of professionals. The most important of these are the Department of Health, the NHS Management Executive (NHSME), the various Regional Health Authorities and, for nurses, the UKCC.

Department of Health circulars and notices are an

important source of information on implementing legislation in the NHS. For example, HN(90)27 and its associated booklet give advice on the removal of crown immunity from the NHS as a result of the NHS and Community Care Act 1990 (Department of Health 1990). Although not having the power of law and, therefore, not resulting in the possibility of any successful criminal or civil action, these guidelines describe good practice and should therefore be accorded due weight. Similarly, the NHSME, on behalf of the Department of Health, brings out at intervals documents commenting on various legal situations and advising NHS bodies on possible action. In the accompanying circular to *A Guide to Consent for Examination or Treatment* (NHSME 1990), there was a requirement for hospitals to respond to the Department of Health on what action they were taking on amending their consent forms. Although sample forms were included in the booklet, there was no requirement that these forms should be adopted.

Circulars and notices issued by individual Regional Health Authorities tend to provide a further supplement to Department of Health and NHSME material. At this level, consultation is more likely than at departmental level, as guidelines are becoming more detailed and only a step away from the organisation producing its own rules and policies. The Data Protection Act 1984 resulted in the production of guidelines at all these levels.

The aims of these guidelines seem to be to assist NHS organisations in interpreting the law and developing good practice. A difficulty in actioning some of these guidelines is the cost implications. A legal requirement *must* be implemented, although the words 'as is reasonable' tend to appear regularly in legal material, with, not surprisingly, a fairly minimal interpretation when resources are scarce. Guidelines, if their implementation beyond the basic legal requirement costs money, are more likely to be set aside or only partially actioned.

While this comment may appear cynical, there seems to be some evidence that NHS organisations have in the past only become responsive to implementing good practice when legal action is taken against them (Rogers and Salvage 1988) or the Health Service Commissioner publishes a report of a complaint adversely affecting them. With NHS Trusts now being responsible for their own costs and any compensation awarded against them arising from court cases (Tingle 1991), the situation has changed to some extent. Trusts are more eager to prevent legal action, and encouraging good practice can achieve this end.

From the nurses' point of view, the underlying reason for promoting good practice may not seem important, but a knowledge of Department of Health and NHSME circulars can provide additional pressure to improve care.

The other source of guidelines on nursing practice is the UKCC. Such material is often published after consultation with national bodies. The importance of the document *The Scope of Professional Practice* (UKCC 1992b) is discussed further later in this chapter, but it is worth noting that it replaced an earlier DHSS circular (DHSS 1977), and the Department of Health (1992) ratified its agreement of this UKCC document. Other guidelines have not always been so well received. A recent statement of the nurses' responsibility regarding their own or colleagues' HIV status has provoked controversy, and it seems likely that many professionals will ignore the advice it contains (UKCC 1992c).

Finally, those nurses who are members of professional bodies and unions may well receive guidelines on relevant and important issues. The authority of these documents is limited but they may in turn be used to influence the UKCC or the Department of Health to produce further guidelines on good practice. The professional can play a part in influencing practice by commenting on proposals put to the membership and becoming active in the policy-forming groups of these organisations.

Rewards and Sanctions

Rewards

The use of rewards to shape behaviour is based on reinforcement theory (Torrington and Hall 1991) and can be applied to the employment arena. In this context, rewards are often limited to financial benefits, but this is a restrictive approach that fails to appreciate what motivates professionals to give of their best.

Rewards can be described as extrinsic or intrinsic. Extrinsic rewards are those related to the general employment context and include pay and conditions of employment. Intrinsic rewards are linked to job content and design. Although extrinsic rewards can assist in recruitment of good staff, it is the intrinsic rewards of the job itself that seem to motivate people to perform well. Job design that encourages autonomy of decision-making and working in teams seems to be particularly valued by professionals, and recognition of achievement through both formal and informal systems is seen as encouraging enthusiasm and commitment (Young 1993).

For nurses there are many intrinsic rewards inherent in the job, and these can be enhanced by managers in a number of ways. Encouraging decision-making through a team approach and enabling individuals to participate in standard-setting will be rewarding to professionals as well as being more likely to lead to improved care.

Of the extrinsic rewards, pay is the most important as it provides a means of social positioning over and above its pure financial value (Brown 1989). The freedom of NHS Trusts to set their own pay levels outside Whitley Council standards, and the implementation of performance-related pay for nurse managers, can be useful but must be viewed with some caution as to their effect on performance and, therefore, patient care.

Sanctions

Sanctions, the other side of the coin from rewards, can be used to control or influence behaviour.

Discipline and dismissal are the ultimate sanctions against unwanted behaviour, but there are many other lesser variants, some of which are the opposite of what nurses find rewarding. Exclusion from decision-making groups and failure to recognise achievement are sanctions that may control some behaviour in the short term but in the long term will tend to reinforce behaviour that is not truly useful to the organisation, ie passivity and an unwillingness to develop new skills. Failure to gain promotion or move sideways into new and challenging jobs is also viewed as a sanction by individuals.

It is not so much the sanctions themselves but the fear of sanctions that creates a powerful effect on behaviour. Nurses will often express helplessness in improving patient care because this will involve speaking out. There is a common perception that such action will be unpopular and result in victimisation, whether or not this is actually the case. There has been much publicity of the issue of 'whistleblowing' (see Chapter 3, *Conflicts of Interest* in this series). For an organisation to overcome this fear of sanctions, it needs to work hard on building an atmosphere of trust rather than suspicion, in which such fears can thrive.

Nevertheless, there is no doubt that a range of sanctions is used to influence behaviour. The bottom line should be whether such sanctions are effective in improving patient care or are being used merely to gain compliance with current authority patterns.

The Influence of Control Mechanisms on Some Key Areas of Nursing

Changing care settings

Over the last few years there has been a major shift in care from the hospital setting into the community. Long-term institutional care has not provided the most appropriate environment for many mentally ill and elderly people and those with learning difficulties. Relocating these individuals in small community houses is now the norm. Length of stay in acute units has been reduced by a rising proportion of day cases and earlier discharge. Such approaches need a shift of resources as well as the development of new skills.

This pattern is having a major impact on the nursing profession. One of the most important documents giving guidance in this area is the UKCC's *The Scope of Professional Practice* (1992b). It states:

> Practice takes place in a context of continuing change and development. Such change and development may result from advances in research leading to improvement in treatment and care, from alterations to the provision of health and social care services, as a result of changes in local policies and as a result of new approaches to professional practice. Practice must, therefore, be sensitive, relevant and responsive to the needs of the individual patients and clients and have the capacity to adjust, where and when appropriate, to changing circumstances.

This document states in effect that each practitioner is personally accountable for her or his own practice and for the maintenance and development of knowledge and competence. This puts the responsibility on the nurse when undertaking new tasks and practising in new areas, and this is supported by a Department of Health (1992) letter, which draws attention to the UKCC's document.

The legal framework also influences nursing practice in changing care settings, the law of negligence being important. If nurses choose to undertake new tasks, they become liable for any errors. However, as long as they are working within their contractual role, the employer will take some responsibility through vicarious liability (Pannett 1992).

Nurses may feel pressured in these situations where they are expected to take on additional responsibilities. It is vitally important that they do not react inappropriately to pressure. As is stated clearly in the Code of Professional Conduct, 'you must . . . acknowledge any limitations in your knowledge and competence and decline any duties or responsibilities unless able to perform them in a safe and skilled manner'. The Wilsher case (*Wilsher* v. *Essex AHA*, 1986–88) reinforced the principle that inexperience can never be an excuse for negligence (Tingle 1988).

Clearly, the UKCC supports the acceptance of nurses' roles changing, and it would be shortsighted of nurses not to ask for or accept these changes. What is crucial is that nursing practice is underpinned by the proper knowledge and skill. Training and education are, therefore, central to enabling nurses to give the care required.

Nurse education has never been a one-off event, but recent and current changes reinforce the continuing nature of learning. Project 2000, as incorporated in the Nurses Rules (Statutory Instruments 1989), puts a much greater emphasis on health and care in the community, while the Post Registration Education and Practice Project (PREPP; UKCC 1991) recommends statutory updating of nurses in order for them to remain on the Register.

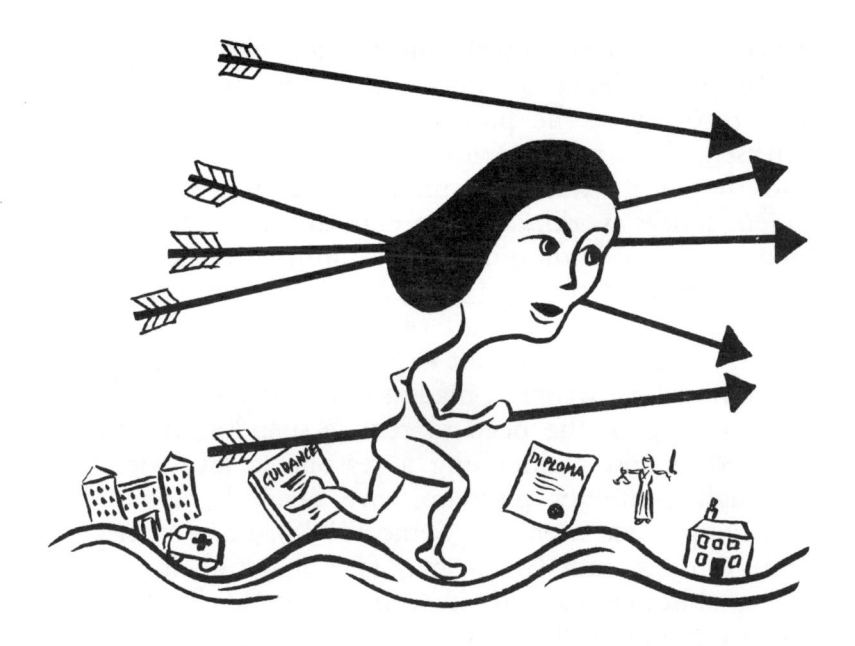

However, as seems to be a common feature of many organisations in the UK during recession (Keep 1989), the training and education budget in the NHS is being squeezed by the current financial problems that most NHS Trusts face. It may well be that the training and education of nurses will be kept at a fairly minimal level in order to reduce costs. Such an approach may simply provide the skills required in the short term but not necessarily the flexibility and motivation that will continue to be needed in the future.

How many nurses?

A continuing problem for nurse managers is the assessment of how many nurses are required and, further, what particular breakdown of skill mix is appropriate.

With a large proportion of the NHS budget being spent on nursing salaries, there is considerable pressure to reduce costs by cutting down on the number and grades of nurses. In spite of evidence to show that patients make a more rapid recovery as the proportion of registered nurses is increased, there is never going to be sufficient money to fund the ideal. With the reduction in the number of student nurses working in the clinical areas, many registered nurses are finding increasing numbers of health care assistants trained to varying NVQ (National Vocational Qualifications) levels as part of the workforce. Numbers of nurses are also being cut as shift patterns are changed and minimal allowance is made for any absence.

For managers, the need to reduce spending has to be balanced against maintaining a reasonable level of care. Although computer program have been developed for forecasting nurse numbers (Senior 1988), nurse managers who get their sums wrong may face an action for negligence, although to date it seems more likely that the practitioners are still the ones carrying the can when mistakes occur. However, managers have been criticised in the arena of the UKCC Professional Conduct Committee for a failure to maintain adequate staff levels.

Part of the professional socialisation process through which new nurses pass inculcates the importance of being seen to cope. Add to that the high value that nurses put on doing their best for their patients and the scene is set for nurses to push themselves beyond the point at which safe care can be assured. As already pointed out, the law on negligence requires only a reasonable level of care, but nurses are usually emotionally driven to excellence and become frustrated at having to accept less.

The Code of Professional Conduct requires nurses to 'report to an appropriate person or authority' their concerns about standards. Legally, this is also important to protect the individual in case mistakes occur as a result of insufficient staff or inappropriate skill mix. In order to ensure that they have evidence of their concerns, nurses would be wise to make any comments in front of a witness and, if their concerns continue, to put the matter in writing to their managers. Fears of victimisation can be more than balanced by fears of possible legal action as a result of negligence. In addition, a manager cannot act without information of potential hazards.

The issue of scarce resources is increasingly ending up in the civil courts. In *Bull and Another v. Devon AHA*, 1989 (Tingle 1990), negligence was proved, but the cause was identified as resources being stretched beyond their limits. Although no blame was attached to specific individuals, the Health Authority was required to pay hefty damages.

Misconduct

A nurse's misconduct could result in a number of outcomes. If the offence is a crime, a nurse could be prosecuted in a criminal court. Penalties for a guilty verdict vary from fines to imprisonment. In addition, the police have a duty to report any successful prosecution of a nurse to the UKCC.

Under civil law, a breach of a nurse's duty of care could lead to him or her being sued. As mentioned, if the wrong occurred during the course and as part of the nurse's employment, the employer will often be sued instead of the nurse, due to vicarious liability. The employer would legally be entitled to claim back any damages from the nurse, but this is rarely, if ever, done.

Of greater immediacy to the nurse is the possible employment outcome of misconduct. The frameworks used arise from legislation, codes of conduct, Whitley Council conditions of employment and local policies. The use of discipline will vary, not only with the actual detail in the local rules, but also with the decisions made by the nurse's immediate manager at the time. Decisions to proceed with disciplinary action may, therefore, be inconsistent, and it is important that those having the responsibility of disciplining staff are properly trained and advised.

All local rules will describe varying levels of disciplinary action, from informal warnings through formal action to dismissal. Essential to any disciplinary action once it reaches the formal stage is the right of appeal.

The involvement of the UKCC in a nurse's misconduct may occur following a criminal conviction or on the nurse's being reported to the UKCC by a member of staff or the public. The UKCC has a legal responsibility to protect the public from unsafe practitioners, which it does through special committees. Allegations of misconduct are investigated and considered by the Preliminary Hearings Committee. This committee may decide to take no action or report the nurse to the Health Committee (if the reason for the misconduct may be due to ill health) or the Professional Conduct Committee.

The law defines misconduct as 'conduct unworthy of a nurse' (Nurses, Midwives and Health Visitors Act 1979), and the standard against which a nurse's performance is judged is the Code of Professional Conduct. The level of proof required by the Professional Conduct Committee is similar to that of a court of law. If misconduct is proved, the committee has several options: no action, administering a formal caution, suspension from the Register or removal from the Register.

One incident of misconduct could, of course, result in several outcomes. It is important that decisions are made as to the appropriate actions to take following an incident of misconduct. To rely on others stepping in because of a personal unwillingness to pursue difficult actions is bad practice. For example, if misconduct should lead to dismissal, it is unacceptable to expect the UKCC to take the matter out of the manager's hands by removing the individual's name from the Register. The nature of proof required by civil, criminal and professional cases may also be different, and the nurse will not have the necessary knowledge to be able to predict the likely outcomes.

Although loyalty to colleagues is a valued characteristic, responsibility towards patients and clients must be the key guiding influence on the nurse's decisions where a workmate is suspected of misconduct.

Conclusion — Control Versus Autonomy

This chapter has taken as its theme the control of professional behaviour. Various methods of control and influence have been explored within the context of nursing practice and patient care.

There is no doubt that the control of human behaviour creates an ethical dilemma. However, the dilemma must be seen in the wider context of both the desirability of certain behaviour and the various possible forms of control that can be used (Kelman 1970).

The desirability of the behaviour begs the question, 'desirable to whom?' Presumably, if the individual seemingly being manipulated has consented to the controls being exercised, this reduces any immorality. Consent presupposes knowledge and understanding, and, as shown in this chapter, the range of control being so wide, the extent of consent may be limited to the democratic right to vote for a detailed involvement in decision-making in the workplace. The inevitability of control in human affairs can be strongly argued, and nurses will, therefore, inevitably be a part of this social phenomenon. It seems likely that control has to be accepted but should not be exercised for the selfish purpose of the controller.

Of the various methods of control and influence described, some can be seen as supportive of good nursing practice, others less so. On the whole, legal controls and professional codes provide broad frameworks in which practice takes place. Individual interpretation is still necessary. Even with the detailed rules developed locally, some discretion in their operation is usually found. The least clearly formulated controls are likely to be the rewards and sanctions operated within organisations, and the very informality of these can lead to unwanted effects.

Two conclusions can be reached as to the scope of the individual practitioner within these frameworks.

Firstly, many nurses have difficulty in coping with uncertainty. Although valuing independence and freedom of choice, the broad frameworks provided often result in the nurse demanding more detail regarding specific application. Surely the underpinning of professional autonomy is an ability and willingness by professionals to make responsible decisions from these guidelines in relation to their own practice. A requirement for such autonomy is knowledge and understanding of the issues. Thus educated practitioners become increasingly important in promoting and maintaining good standards of care.

The second issue relates to reducing the manipulative aspects of control mechanisms at a personal level. The first step needs to be an awareness of one's own values, followed by consciously minimising the effect of these when influencing others. This should enable the person being influenced to exercise a wider range of choices within constraints that are unavoidable. Whether a nurse is functioning as a manager, a team member or a practitioner, the resulting way of working with subordinates, colleagues, patients or clients has within it the seeds of encouraging a climate of individual responsibility within the controls of professional behaviour.

References

Bowers, J (1990) *Bowers on Employment Law.* London: Blackstone Press.
Brown, W (1989) Managing remuneration, In Sisson, K (ed.), *Personnel Management in Britain.* Oxford: Blackwell.
Department of Health (1990) *Removal of Crown Immunities.* HN(90)27. London: Department of Health.
Department of Health (1992) *The Extended Role of the Nurse/Scope of Professional Practice.* PL/CNO (92)4. London: Department of Health.
DHSS (1977) *The Extending Role of the Clinical Nurse — Legal Implications and Training Requirements.* HC(77)22. London: DHSS.
Dimond, B (1990) *Legal Aspects of Nursing.* London: Prentice Hall.
Dwan, S (1992) *The 'commercial venture' Requirement in the Transfer Regulations.* Crown's Employer's Briefing No. 25.
Dyer, C (1992) Case to stop food 'overwhelming'. *The Guardian*, 20 Nov., p. 2.
Handy, C (1985) *Gods of Management* (revised edn.). London: Pan Books.
International Council for Nurses (1973) *Code for Nurses.* Geneva: ICN.
Keep, E (1989) A training scandal?, In Sisson, K (ed.), *Personnel Management in Britain*, pp. 177–82. Oxford: Blackwell.
Kelman, HC (1970) Manipulation of human behaviour: an ethical dilemma for the social scientist, In Bennis, WG, Benn, KD and Chin R (eds), *The Planning of Change* (2nd edn.). London: Holt, Rinehart and Winston.
Mason, JK and McCall Smith, RA (1987) *Law and Medical Ethics* (2nd edn.). London: Butterworth.
National Back Pain Association (1992) *The Guide to the Handling of Patients* (3rd edn.). London: NBPA and RCN.
National Health Service and Community Care Act (1990). London: HMSO.
NHS Management Executive (1990) *A Guide to Consent for*

Examination or Treatment. London: NHSME, Department of Health.
Nurses, Midwives and Health Visitors Act (1979). London: HMSO.
Padfield, C (1983) *Law Made Simple*. (Revised by FE Smith, 6th edn.). London: Heinemann.
Pannett, AJ (1992) *Law of Torts* (6th edn.). London: Pitman.
Rogers, R and Salvage, J (1988) *Nurses at Risk: A Guide to Health and Safety at Work*. London: Heinemann.
Salvage, J (1985) *The Politics of Nursing*. London: Heinemann.
Senior, OE (1988) Manpower planning objectives and information systems, In Hudson, D (ed.), *Recent Advances in Nursing: Nursing Administration*. Edinburgh: Churchill Livingstone.
Skegg, PDG (1984) *Law, Ethics & Medicine*. Oxford: Clarendon Press.
Statutory Instruments (1989) *The Nurses, Midwives and Health Visitors (Training) Amendment Rules Approval Order No. 1456*. London: HMSO.
Tingle, JH (1988) Negligence and Wilsher. *Solicitors Journal*, **132**(25): 910–11.
Tingle, JH (1990) The important case of Bull. *Nursing Standard*, **4**(37): 54–5.
Tingle, JH (1991) Who pays for clinical negligence? *New Law Journal*, May 10, 630–50.
Torrington, D and Hall, L (1991) *Personnel Management* (2nd edn.). London: Prentice Hall.
UKCC (1986) *Project 2000: A New Preparation for Practice*. London: UKCC.
UKCC (1987) *Confidentality*. London: UKCC.
UKCC (1989) *Exercising Accountability*. London: UKCC.
UKCC (1990) Statement on advertising and commercial sponsorship. London: UKCC.
UKCC (1991) *PREPP and You*. London: UKCC.
UKCC (1992a) *Code of Professional Conduct* (3rd edn.). London: UKCC.
UKCC (1992b) *The Scope of Professional Practice*. London: UKCC.
UKCC (1992c) *AIDS and HIV Infection*. London: UKCC.

UKCC (1993) *The Council's Proposed Standards for Post-Registration Education.* London: UKCC.
Young, AP (1989) *Legal Problems in Nursing Practice.* London: Chapman and Hall.
Young, AP (1993) The use of rewards for employees in the NHS. *Journal of Nursing Management,* **2**: 177–83.
Young, AP (1994) *Law and Professional Conduct in Nursing* (2nd edn.). London: Scutari Press.

CHAPTER 3
Standards of Practice
Betty Kershaw

> Standards of practice, like personal and social values, change constantly. This is not only a threat to a profession, but also its main challenge.
>
> Students come to nursing with their own luggage of values and points of references, and they quickly have to learn to accept the new ways and values of their patients and clients, and also their colleagues and employers. However, they also have to learn to challenge them and question them, not in order to destroy them or ridicule them, but in order to enhance their ethical practice and care.
>
> This chapter addresses a great many of these issues in the very practical way that characterises the author's particular contribution to nursing.

Nurses have always been concerned from a personal and professional perspective about standards of practice. We, as nurses, have always striven to give the highest possible care and have constantly adapted care-giving to meet the changes others demanded or we demanded of ourselves. We have seen nursing continue to hold public confidence in our standards of care through the demise of the matron in the 1960s, the introduction of the Salmon Management initiative of the 1970s, general management of the 1980s and now NHS Trusts. In some instances, Trust management has strengthened the nursing voice by appointing nurse managers as Trust nurses, even entitling the post-holder 'Matron', but in other instances nursing has lost its managers.

However, managers manage nurses and nursing; they do not lead it. Management and leadership are fundamentally different skills, and only the very ablest demonstrate competence in both. Managers regulate the climate in which care is given and manage those who deliver the service. Nurse managers must face the major professional conflicts of the 1990s as they strive to manage the service and to maintain and improve standards of practice and quality of care within a climate of constant change and an almost permanent cost improvement programme. Their work is not always helped by the increasing demands of practising nurses for the means to introduce new research findings, nursing developments and practice changes, which are being written and spoken about and, indeed, implemented by nursing leaders at all levels.

This chapter aims to explore these changes and how they have affected standards of practice as we know them today. It will discuss personal and professional conflict and address the debates about the situation at present, the ethical framework within which care is delivered and the trends that appear to be shaping the future.

Debates on the quality of care, nursing and medical ethics, professional practice, efficiency and effectiveness, increasing numbers of patients being treated, 'whistleblowing', politics (and the political framework within which care is delivered), financing the NHS and the social structure of present-day society have been prominent within the national and nursing press throughout the last decade. The situation has been complicated by the introduction of NHS Trusts, fund-holding general practitioners and private medicine, and the different way in which patients and clients are treated depending on how the costs of that treatment are to be met.

The comfortable, care-orientated framework for practice within which nursing has operated for a century and a half is in danger (some would see this already as a reality) of being lost within the competitive, challenging world of health care economics of today. Such a framework is based on the tenet of Nightingale (1859) 'to do the sick no harm' and Henderson's (1966) statement, 'the unique function of the nurse is to assist the patient, sick or well, in the performance of those activities of daily living which they would perform unaided had they the necessary strength, will or knowledge'. Nurses have felt comfortable with these expressions, which encompass the skilled caring role within which they feel secure.

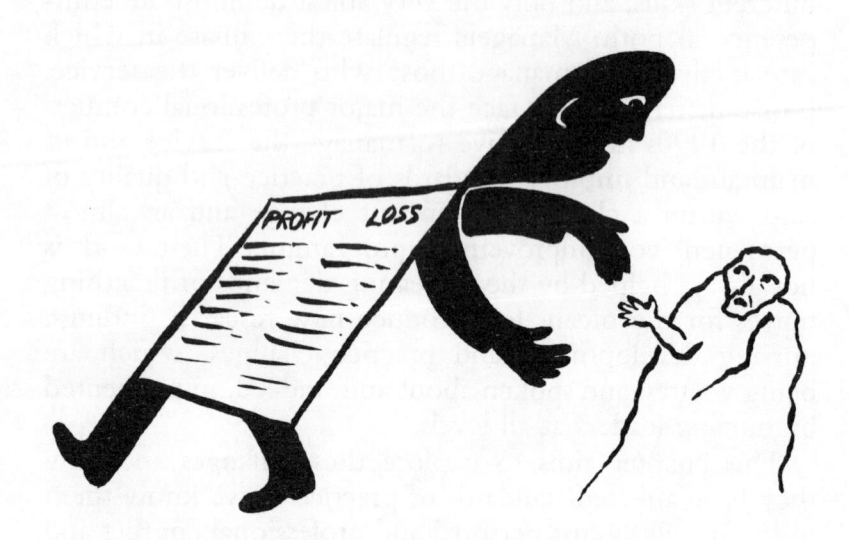

As we move through the last decade of the 20th century, this approach to care is constantly challenged. Nursing is now being increasingly compared to a conveyor belt job, where patients and staff are manipulated and moved like objects, and within which standard or uniform care and treatment is seen as the order of the day.

- I trained as a general nurse in the early 1960s in a large, acute, medical-school-linked general hospital where the baseline for our practice was professional loyalty, respect for tradition and subservience to the decisions made and directions given by senior nurses and doctors (Salvage 1985). The unquestionable obedience saved us from considerable ethical conflict (after all were not those dual 'gods' always right?) and the unwavering routine ensured that we always knew what to do. We could always measure it 'having been done' very accurately too. One merely ticked the work book. Our ethical code of the day followed the Nightingale approach in that we looked to doctors for direction and reflected the Hippocratic Oath in that we too 'did the sick no harm'. I remember being presented with the International Council of Nurses (ICN) Code of Ethics, but remember no discussion or debate about it, nor it being referred to ever again.

Conflict

Inherent in this approach to the profession's ethical behaviour was the ostracism of those who began to question ('criticise' would be too strong a word) and the isolation they began to experience from professional colleagues. Gillon (1985) acknowledges this in discussing medical ethics, and Salvage (1985) raises issues reflecting this in relation to nursing. It seems that not much has changed. Why else would so many nurses write to the press with negative points or comments requesting that their names should not be published?

But the right, indeed the duty, to criticise and question is now coming to the fore of professional practice. The Royal College of Nursing's public forum for debate (Congress) has debated 'whistleblowing' on several occasions, the most recent being in 1993 (RCN 1993) when the issue was set within the framework of the UKCC's 1992 edition of the Code of Professional Conduct (UKCC 1992a). The question centred on what nurses should do next when, having followed the Code in the interest of patient care and complained to those responsible, they find no action being taken.

There is no need to look any further for an area of concern to nurses, wherever they work, than this. The election of Graham Pink to the 1993 UKCC Executive Council (from which he has now resigned) showed how closely nurses empathise with this problem and how much they want an answer. This is the question that will direct ethical debate in the 1990s as nurses try to maintain quality of delivery and standards of practice.

The Royal College of Nursing has called for a managers' code of conduct. It said that 'such a code would act as a set of guidance for managers and help demonstrate the values they share with clinical staff' (Turner 1994).

One vehicle for addressing the conflict for nurses who feel that their standards are being compromised was issued by the UKCC in the autumn of 1992 (UKCC 1992b). This letter, and the set of standards attached, immediately threw into the public arena the ethical conflict between professional nurses working as purchasers and those who are responsible for health care delivery. The first statement in the set of standards reminds nurses of 'The Council's legally prescribed duties and its Code of Professional Conduct':

> The Council regulates the nursing, midwifery and health visiting professional in the interests of public protection and in order to secure standards of care which are at least safe for patients and clients.

There is no doubt that this published support from the UKCC has been long awaited in that it moves the debate about ethics and nursing into the new area of public conflict. No longer can professionally qualified managers and teachers make statements about standards of practice and then not take steps to monitor whether these standards are achieved and, when necessary, facilitate that achievement.

The debate, recognising the conflict between efficiency and nursing ethics, is ably summarised by Chadwick and Tadd (1992), who suggest that major elements in a contract should include patient safety, respect for patient dignity and speed of response to requests for treatment, care and services, and that these are quality measures frequently used to document improvement in the quality of care. They dispute, as do many nurses, that mere measurement of standards being achieved is in itself quality. But the measurement of some quality standards is easier to address than others. As nurses, we need to ensure that we do not compromise our personal ethical code by complacently accepting the achievement of those standards that are easily quantifiable (for example increased patient throughput and reduced waiting time) without looking at the practices behind the figures.

Practice and education have moved rapidly since the 1960s, and the ethical behaviour of nurses is addressed and directed in the UKCC Code of Professional Conduct. The battle for professional ethical standards has been a long one and is by no means over. A brief review of the literature on this topic demonstrates a history of the fight only too well. *Sans Everything* (Robb 1967) was perhaps the first publication to address the issue of students complaining about care, in this case care being given to patients in a large psychiatric hospital. This led to the first of several government enquiries into standards of nursing care. Salvage (1985) documents the stance taken by nurses refusing on ethical grounds to take part in electroconvulsive therapy (ECT). She also records the 1984 'Nurse Alert' campaign, which was monitored by the Royal College of Nursing (RCN). This project asked nurses to highlight falling standards of care. More recently (1992), the RCN has had to set up a confidential telephone line to help nurses who are having conflicts with their professional ethics and are being asked to compromise them.

However one views the conflict between managers and nurses, there is no doubt that it is increasing and is causing distress to both. The gap between NHS Management (at national and local level) and personal and professional ethics would seem to be widening. Chadwick and Tadd (1992) remind us that the underlying 'principles of medical ethics — autonomy, beneficence, non-maleficence and justice — are equally applicable to nursing'. They question, however, whether they can be applied within the 'market-orientated health care service'. There are many nurses who would agree with them: it is the application of ethical standards that forms the kingpin of the UKCC's Registrar's 1992 letter. In seeking to address how far this advice is realistic and relevant to present-day practice, one needs to move forward by exploring some of the issues facing student nurses where the Project 2000 (UKCC 1986) curriculum is encouraging them to address ethics, professional growth and legal issues.

Firstly, students are taught that it is important to recognise the legislative framework that gives strength to the UKCC Code of Professional Conduct; it is equally important to recognise that moral and philosophical issues are above the law — inasmuch as there can be 'bad laws'. Gillon (1985) summarises the ethical Declarations of the World Medical Association. He makes it quite clear that medical knowledge must not be used 'contrary to the laws of humanity' and enjoins doctors to recognise that the Declarations of their world body contain a considerable number of moral guidelines which 'purport to govern medical practice'.

Not only do legislation and our knowledge of it underlie our ethical principles but so do our culture, socialisation, religious understanding and practice and personal experiences. A frequently cited example is the legislation surrounding abortion in England and Wales. Abortion within certain circumstances is lawful, but some groups find this difficult to accept. Societies where children are seen as one's investment for the future (in that infant mortality rates have been so high one needed several sons for one to be kept comfortable in old age) tend to continue with a high birth rate in the UK. They are reluctant to use contraception and equally reluctant to accept abortion when the fetus is likely (or known) to be damaged. The Roman Catholic Church bans abortion; the young girl who is not a Catholic herself but who attended a Catholic school, has Catholic friends (or who is just questioning religion) may well be socialised into that point of view. Personal experiences also influence choice. Friends and families colour how we view our own ethical perspectives of life and influence the decisions we make. One of the first lessons nursing students have to learn is how to integrate their own experiences with those of their patients and clients and how to address differing values constructively.

The 'Right to Know'

One way to be able to have the 'right to know' is to ensure that all decisions are made with 'informed consent', which Gillett (1989) defines as 'the principle that a person has a right to make free and informed decisions about what happens to her'. Gillett recognises that consent can be explicit or implicit but stresses that consent must be given if at all possible. As long ago as 1967, Ley and Spelman's research study explored the information that doctors gave patients and families and what they remembered of it. They found that patients remembered very little of what was said, and that what they did remember was either the good news, information which reinforced what they thought themselves or 'very bad news'. Generally, alternative or education information was forgotten. Their findings are very relevant for today's settings where it is known that stress inhibits even very positive events and how we hear and perceive them.

Ways of ensuring that patients have assistance in making choices for informed consent are to offer the opportunity for a friend or relative to listen and participate and to provide follow-up written material for patients to take and read in their own time. A third way is to ensure that the patient's primary or named nurse is present if possible, which enables the matter discussed to be reinforced.

In giving information to patients, one must beware of patronising and of speaking down (or up), and one must check to make sure that the patient and relatives understand the information. This is especially important when the family speak little English and even more so when one has to rely on an interpreter. The story is told of a nurse who works in a Muslim country and frequently comments on male interpreters who, when working with female patients, do not ask the questions which are 'of a female nature' but make up the answers, whether true or not. There is no way of knowing how accurate the story is, but it does counsel us to remember to provide information booklets and leaflets in appropriate languages.

Tied in with the ethical issue of informed consent is the whole framework of patient information and the individual's right to know. The Access to Health Records Act 1990 is now in force, but a Private Member's Bill was tabled in the House of Commons in February 1993 that aimed to increase further the access patients have to their medical records. Doctors can restrict access to information if they consider that that information would harm the patient; such information may concern diagnosis, treatment outcome or mental state, for example. One of the areas in which nurses and doctors conflict is the knowledge which a patient should have about a terminal prognosis. Nurses frequently maintain that patients should be given the information about their treatment options, care, etc. and decide who should be party to that information. Increasingly, nurses are facing ethical conflict when doctors insist that patients are not told a diagnosis, but their relatives are, the latter then being forced to play a 'secrecy game' (Ellis and Hartley 1988). MP Mark Fisher's Bill opens this debate by bringing such conflicts onto the public floor of the House of Commons.

Advocacy

Other conflicting issues which are often raised in debate on ethical matters include decision-making about treatment for children and those who have a diagnosed long-term mental illness or are known to have a substantial learning difficulty, often with additional physical handicap. Chadwick and Tadd (1992) note the growing interest in advocacy for patients, especially the mentally ill. Advocacy is recognised in law, but any nurse planning to introduce it into her or his nursing practice would be well advised to take the counsel of Chadwick and Tadd who suggest caution. This is offered on the grounds of lack of knowledge of law and its application and, of course, on the stress involved. The UKCC's Code of Professional Conduct (1992a) also recognises advocacy. It is seen there as 'promoting and safe-guarding the wellbeing and interests of patients', with less emphasis on the legal aspects of the role of nurses.

The issues of law and ethics are constantly intermingling, intermixing and conflicting. Gillon (1985) cites at length the arguments for and against what is known as the Arthur case: 'In November 1981 a respected physician, the late Dr Leonard Arthur, was acquitted of the attempted murder of a newborn infant with Down's Syndrome for whom he prescribed dihydrocodeine and 'nursing care only' after the baby had been rejected by his mother'. Gillon refers to the case for the prosecution and the defence. The arguments are not new, but are well summarised. They revolve around all life being equal, about the duty of care laid on doctors, about the obligation to 'do the sick no harm' and about equality under the law. One could also, as others have done, remind readers of the euthanasia programmes of Nazi Germany. The debate moves on to whether, if one can withdraw support from a baby who is rejected and handicapped, one can do it to (and for, if one believes in the 'quality of life' argument) any older mentally handicapped or mentally ill person who is also rejected.

The case for the defence concentrates on the quality of life arguments, on the Hippocratic Oath and on the duty of care — but viewed from different angles and perspectives. The central conclusion of the 'defence' appears to be concentrated on the understanding that although the doctor should not harm those for whom he or she has a duty of care, 'he is not obliged in all circumstances to prevent the patient dying'.

The case of Tony Bland, the young man injured in the Hillsborough stadium disaster and left in a persistent vegetative state for nearly four years, had several similarities to and differences from 'baby X' in the Arthur case. The similarities lie in the parents' wish for life to end, in doctors supporting this wish and in the 'seen' public support. *The Daily Telegraph* editorial of February 5th 1993 openly states (of the Tony Bland case): 'few will doubt that the decision ... was compassionate and right'. The editorial continues to raise the issue of 'old law, new medicine', an issue which we will return to later, since it is very relevant to the Code of Professional Conduct (1992a) with which nurses work today.

'Old Law, New Medicine'

The Tony Bland case is not the first case of ethical issues which has challenged legality at the highest level, but it is one of the few in which nurses' interests are mentioned, and where nursing and medical ethics can conflict.

At the time of the Arthur case, senior nurses debated the issue in the national press, comparing the case with other quality of life and equal access cases such as patients with spina bifida or a need for kidney transplantation. Curiously, none of this public debate was addressed in any of the 'locatable' literature on the case. It was as if the doctors, and the doctors alone, had ethical considerations for practice.

Before we explore the Tony Bland case any further, it is timely to return to the 'old law, new medicine' debate. *The Daily Telegraph*, in its editorial on February 5th 1993, quite rightly points out that legislators in the case had to make logical decisions 'at a level of abstraction far removed from the reality of scientific intensive care'. Included in this interpretation must also be the intensive care regimes and invasive procedures that carry life-support systems. What, yet again, is not mentioned is the skilled nursing and therapist care and intervention. None of the reports of that day mentioned the nursing ethics involved and none debated the ethical basis from which therapists practise. Doctors hold the legal 'duty of care', and it is doctors who were seen to make the decisions. We hear from Tony's parents, who quite rightly had a major voice in the care their son received, but not from those who cared for him on a day-to-day, hour-by-hour basis. Perhaps they were called to discuss Tony Bland's future, but if so, it is sad that one did not see the reports of their opinions on the case.

Dr Howe, the physician treating Tony Bland, supported the decision (to withdraw nourishment and so let Tony Bland die) in a letter to *The Guardian* on February 10th 1993. He cited his own research into similar cases in the USA and Canada (where patients in a persistent vegetative state [PVS] are not actively treated), the judgements of their legislators and the opinions of the British Medical Association (BMA). Dr Howe asks 'can such an existence have any human value?' and continues to say that 'to maintain such an existence is cruel and stupid'.

The arguments to support his case from a medical perspective are persuasive and have sense on their side. Their ethical and legal values have been upheld — as a medical decision. Whether they are upheld as a nursing decision is still open to debate.

For many years, nurses have recognised that when medical intervention is unsuccessful and the patient is seen to be dying, the role of the nurse becomes paramount. Patients for whom there is no hope of recovery are bypassed by medical staff who are seen to lose interest when there is no intervention of theirs that can be successful.

So much of Tony Bland's care until he died on March 3rd 1993 fell on the nurses, and the stress that this would bring them was recognised. The Airedale Hospital staff were offered supportive counselling throughout his dying and beyond. Part of their stress related to the fact that medical and nursing concepts on patient care and treatment differ, especially for dying patients, and our ethical perspectives are, therefore, not always the same.

In a letter to *The Guardian* (February 11th 1993), Stephen Wright, a Fellow of the RCN, a member of its Council and the first consultant nurse in the UK, challenged Dr Howe's assumption on the 'rightness' of the decision. He pointed out that most nurses do not see the use of nasal or oral gastric tubes as medical intervention but as an essential form of life support. He stated that the withdrawal of Tony Bland's feeding tube confronted nurses with the most profound moral and ethical dilemma. This is not a case of switching machines to the 'off' position, since Tony Bland breathed by his own respiratory stimulus. Wright also pointed out that there are issues of quality of life involved, in that a patient in a persistent vegetative state is unaware and cannot, therefore, have a quality of life to lose. Since he is not 'sentient', to quote Wright, he can have no best interests. The interests being served are, therefore, those of others. Wright raised the question of whether ethical values are there for our own benefit or for others, and suggested that there are times when ethical standards certainly do not make nurses more comfortable.

This is especially true when, as in the Tony Bland and the Arthur cases, the nursing and medical staff's ethical perspectives clash. There are, of course, many areas where they are congruent, where they are compatible and where they totally and utterly agree. But individual nurses may stand at opposite ends of the spectrum since each person's ethical values are based on personal socialisation, moral and religious background, nursing (and indeed life) experiences and where one works.

The Nurses' Viewpoint

If we need a reminder of how personal ethics is (Gillon 1985), we have only to consider any student's perspective of nursing ethics. The Project 2000 curricula invariably have a unit, module, theme or thread on nursing ethics, moral issues, professional standards or a similar topic. Students' anxieties over how they 'fit in' over the conflicts they have about standards and values are often raised at student conferences and in the press. Salvage (1985) reminds us that members new to the profession often see issues with new eyes and with the viewpoint of the public, that is the patients or clients for whom they care. In other words, they represent the consumer (to quote the marketplace language of the present health care environment) and can be seen as the patient's advocate. They may indeed be better fitted to fulfil this role in some respects than an experienced nurse who has been socialised into the profession.

Some of the issues raised by nurses time and again are (sadly) very old. Even in this day of *The Patient's Charter* (1991) which clearly states that patients and their families must be consulted about, involved in and receive explanations of, their care, all levels of nurse continue to express anxiety about patients not being told the truth about diagnosis, about medical staff talking to relatives without the patient's permission, using relatives' wishes as an excuse not to address the issue with the patient, and about rendering nurses powerless by forbidding discussion of what they themselves do not wish to discuss.

We also hear of nurses being caught in the conflict between doctors over treatment options. Perhaps the most under-publicised issue (it has since been on television, in the national press and in *Reader's Digest*) is that of treatment options for breast cancer. For over 40 years, the treatment was mastectomy, often radical, followed by extensive radiotherapy and supportive chemotherapy. This 'package' was invasive to the woman's body image, attacking her sexuality, her femininity, her future (Salter 1988). Increasingly, oncologists have recognised alternatives, such as lumpectomy, with correctly balanced supportive treatment such as chemotherapy and radiotherapy, based on individual patient assessment. Repeatedly, we hear of patients who are still not offered choices but whose surgeons make the decisions for them. This inevitably leaves nurses to make excuses and to compromise their own ethical opinions of patient choice in their other ethical obligation of supporting the doctors. How does one justify to a patient and family a decision made without consultation, one which one knows to be out of date, old-fashioned and not based on relevant research?

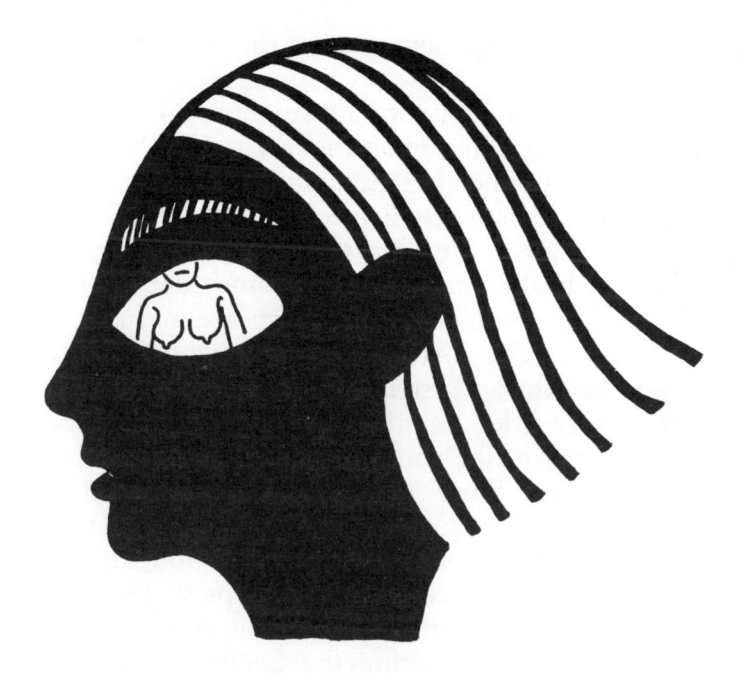

The same can be said about the scepticism poured on the use of massage, aromatherapy or reflexology. Nurses are increasingly wishing to offer such treatments and can produce sound evidence for their reasons. The public at large is increasingly aware of the value of such options; for example, *The Observer* (February 21st 1993) had a full-page article detailing the use of psychotherapy, physiotherapy, occupational therapy and nursing to promote positive pain relief at a holistic clinic that advocates relaxation and teaches it as a means of adapting to intractable pain. How do nurses cope with the ethical dilemmas posed when patients facing increasing drug dependency for pain request such treatment options?

Even more so, in the last two cases, how do they address personal ethical conflict when therapy is available to some patients but not others? This frequently moves on to a debate about private medicine, which seems to offer choice. Most nurses are able to choose whether or not they work in health care that is insurance driven, so they should have no ethical conflict with choice in this context. Much more likely to invoke stress is the conflict between the present health care system and its marketplace perspectives. We heard a lot in the early months of 1993 about access to treatment for patients from fundholding general practitioners and those who were not 'so fortunate'. Where health authorities were the purchasers (and had run out of cash) it seemed impossible for non-urgent care and treatment to be accessed, and the press, in March of that year, began to publish letters about deaths of patients on waiting lists, thus forcing the Secretary of State for Health to review her policy. In 1994, it was the turn in the spotlight of the elderly, who were refused care on the premise that they would no longer benefit from it.

Ethical dilemmas change all the time. Some arise from political decisions, some from new knowledge and some from personal entrenchment against new ideas. Advances in diagnosis bring their own problems, such as when an EMR scanner identifies minute secondaries that were not suspected. Is there a justification for treating the primary tumour when it gives no symptoms? There are those who would argue in favour of this, just as there are those who would suggest that the money would be better spent elsewhere.

Personal Choice

Nurses are constantly being called upon to make decisions that can be seen as ethical. If you have a cold, do you come on duty — thereby ensuring that the staff is at full complement — but risk infecting not only other staff but patients too? If you see a very stressed and overworked colleague being rough rather than gentle, aggressive rather than persuasive, with a confused old lady, do you report him or her or do you accept that this is not his or her usual behaviour and make allowances? What do you do about a blatant lie? For example, an Asian woman requests to see a female doctor, but is told that none is available, even when you know that this is merely a 'convenience' since the female doctor would have to come from another unit. Sometimes it must seem that the whole of the NHS is making excuses for others.

Consider yet another scenario, related to an article in *The Guardian* (March 12th 1993) which is only too familiar to many nurses who have worked in general hospitals over the last 30 or 40 years. This article reported the death of a patient following both her and her husband's refusal for her to have a blood transfusion, because it was against her beliefs as a Jehovah's Witness. How do you feel about this patient dying? The judge stated: 'I find it very difficult to accept the consequences of these beliefs should extend to two children who lost their mother as a result'. The anaesthetist commented, 'I am positive her life would have been saved'. Has a patient the right to refuse treatment? Is that right of refusal different when others are affected by it (in this case the children)? What is your ethical position about the medical staff allowing her to die? There was a time when serious discussion would have centred on whether or not adults, like children, can be made wards of court, or when doctors would have transfused a patient behind the closed doors of the operating theatre and not told anyone. Where would you have stood in that debate?

If one listens to nurses discussing ethics, debating them at RCN Congress or giving seminar presentations, other issues come to the fore: the doctor who 'does a D&C' on every rape victim she examines as a police surgeon just to make sure she aborts any fetus; or the surgeon who sterilises the multiparous mother 'just as part of the section'. These are ethical issues that concern nurses as much as doctors.

In none of these cases could the patient be said to be giving informed consent; neither can they in situations where they are entered into drug trials without knowledge or are fed placebo medication because no one believes their pain.

The present government is trying to open up the debate on informed consent, on patient participation in treatment and on access to records. All this is good, as are the initiatives on resource management, with its strategies of auditing and review. But it will only be as good as the professional bravery in speaking out. Students still report anxiety at acting as an advocate, and very senior staff report the need for facilitators because they fear victimisation. These facilitators are often the editors of nursing journals who will publish letters and raise issues anonymously. It is sad that it has still to be done in this way. Sometimes, such letters will detail how the writers felt unsupported: their ward sister, nurse manager or teacher had failed to become involved and to demonstrate belief in what was happening. This is of course not confined to nurses. *The Observer* (February 21st 1993) documents a long history of disbelief in relation to the use of 'pindown' in social service care centres and of social workers' failure to believe children and young adults who reported abuse. Nurses, too, are not believed when they report their own sexual harassment (Salvage 1985) or that of others in their care (*The Observer*, as above). Students see abuse in many ways: dressing a female elderly confused lady in underpants because there are no knickers; restraining a patient so that medicine can be poured down his throat; the constraints on a patient's mobility when he or she is left in nightclothes all day. Students report anger at staff not recognising their dilemma and anger that the socialisation that staff have gone through has blinded them to the ethical issues as students see them. Often, when such dilemmas are brought into the open, explanations are given — they may not be satisfactory to all concerned, and the sadness is that they need a third party in the first place.

Nurses seem to find it difficult to explain their ethical values of practice or even recognise that they are there. Wright (1990) offers some solutions to this 'blindness' that comes with familiarity — the familiarity that breeds contempt — of values. When writing of introducing change in a clinical environment, he cites several issues that can cause minor ethical conflict. Wright mentions toilets with doors which do not shut (or indeed that have no doors), a lack of choice in diet and drinks, putting patients to bed at 4.00 pm because it is easier for staff, or not dressing patients at all so that they cannot wander. By careful staff relocation and re-education, nurses and nursing assistants have come to view such practices as out of date and realise that they devalue themselves as well as the patient's individuality.

So far, we have explored ethical issues that will be recognised by all nurses, many being confined to the society in which we care. These ethical issues may conflict with law, but do not of themselves seem criminal to many nurses.

Those who disagree with any decision usually see an alternative perspective and can empathise with those (for example Tony Bland's parents) who are deeply troubled by the conflicts they have aroused and the publicity they have created.

Public Issues

However, there are other ethical issues that nurses raise from time to time. Nurses working in Accident and Emergency departments (especially students who may not be involved with active life-saving intervention) mention the difficulty they have in caring for the car driver (perhaps drunk) who has hit a lamp-post and badly injured his passenger.

The ethical conflict aroused as one provides care for the person responsible can take time to adjust to. But if one begins to apportion blame, where does one stop? Is the patient with lung cancer responsible for his own malignancy because he smoked? Is the woman trying to conceive responsible for her own infertility because of the abortion she had when a teenager? Is the man now having a psychiatric crisis due to a family breakdown responsible for that because the breakdown was accelerated through his abuse of his own family?

As health carers we all try hard to be non-judgemental and to treat all patients and clients alike, regardless of our own particular feelings and opinions. Our ethics must be seen to be above reproach. But this becomes increasingly difficult to practise. Within the marketplace of health care today, we are seeing decisions being made as patients are selected for treatment on the basis of age, occupation and responsibilities. Questions are being asked when a 69-year-old person is admitted to an intensive care unit but a 71-year-old is not, and when a working man is said to be given priority for surgery over an unemployed neighbour. Infertility treatment is increasingly only available to those who pay. The whole issue of access and ethics has become an urgent debate.

Similarly, Britain is increasingly becoming a multiethnic society, and nurses are being faced with ethical dilemmas that would have been unknown or impossible to contemplate to those now old enough to be in senior positions. In 1993 a clinic was opened in London that offers amniocentesis to pregnant women. Nothing new about that — many women are offered that facility if it is expected that the fetus they carry could be damaged in some way. While this has its own ethical debate, as does the option of abortion which follows diagnosis, this clinic is not primarily about that. What is being offered is 'sexing', that is identifying at the fetal stage the sex of the fetus. While occasionally a son and heir may be wanted, most patients are happy to have a healthy child. However, Britain is a multiracial society, and there are now cultures within it that see male children as more important. Women who are carrying babies of the 'wrong' sex are at risk of being pressurised by their culture to seek abortion on psychological grounds. The ethics of this could be another debate for the future.

With us already are the issues surrounding female circumcision. On March 3rd 1993, *The Guardian* raised the issue of culture and law and ethics, citing the legislation that is enacted in France to prevent this practice happening. To quote the author, 'health workers fear that 10,000 children (in the UK) are at risk of being excised'. She reminds us that those encouraging it, or indeed practising it, can be subject to prosecution under child abuse legislation and disagrees with those who see it as a cultural issue and a procedure that should be available to those who want it as an aseptic surgical procedure. In France, 10 cases have been brought before the courts since 1988 (*The Guardian* March 3rd 1993), several involving more than one young girl. Four children are known to have died.

Until 1991, the cultural argument had been successful in ensuring that suspended sentences only had been given, but since then courts are sentencing to imprisonment both parents and the person performing the operation. Women's groups, especially nurses and midwives who see the immediate and later trauma resulting from these operations, are beginning to debate the issue and the ethics involved.

There is no doubt that such an operation is abuse and indeed rank cruelty, in that it is usually done without anaesthetic, analgesia or asepsis and puts the child at risk of shock, urine retention, tetanus, blood loss, pelvic infection and HIV as immediate issues, and major infertility and childbirth problems in the future. But if it is only abuse, how does one feel about reports that private clinics are offering the operation as a surgical procedure? This then would not constitute physical abuse — or would it? And is psychological abuse part of the same ethical issue?

Conclusion

Such issues of professional ethics will form ongoing debates. Ethical behaviour is about respecting those for whom we care and about valuing ourselves and our profession. It is about never stopping asking questions when we feel that something is wrong (even if we feign innocence in the approach taken); it is about not failing to support those who come to us for help, about not being compromised, about treating others as we would wish ourselves, our families and our friends to be treated and about believing in nursing and all that it stands for.

Nurses have much respect and love from patients, clients, their families, friends and the public at large. The least we, as nurses, owe the public is to ensure that our own ethical basis for care is above reproach.

References

Chadwick, R and Tadd, W (1992) *Ethics and Nursing Practice*. London: Macmillan.
The Daily Telegraph: Old law, new medicine (February 5th 1993).
Department of Health (1991) *The Patients' Charter*. London: HMSO.
Ellis, JR and Hartley, CL (1988) *Nursing in Today's World: Challenges, Issues and Trends*. Philadelphia, USA: Lippincott and Co.
Gillett, P (1989) *Reasonable Care*. Bristol: Bristol University Press.
Gillon, RF (ed.) (1985) *Philosophical Medical Ethics*. Chichester: John Wiley and Sons.
The Guardian: A time to live and a time to die (February 10th 1993); Ethics and a matter of life and death (February 11th 1993); A knife in any language (March 3rd 1993); Jehovah's Witness dies after refusing blood transfusion (March 12th 1993).
Henderson, V (1966) *The Nature of Nursing*. New York: Macmillan.
Ley, P and Spelman, M (1967) *Communicating with the Patient*. London: Staples Press.
Nightingale, F (1859, re-issued 1980) *Notes on Nursing*. Edinburgh: Churchill Livingstone.
The Observer: Breaking through the pain barrier (February 21st 1993).
RCN (1993) *Congress Agenda 1993*. London: RCN.
Robb, B (1967) *Sans Everything: A Case to Answer*. Walton-on-Thames: Nelson.
Salter, M (1988) *Altered Body Image*. Chichester: John Wiley and Sons.
Salvage, J (1985) *The Politics of Nursing*. London: Heinemann.
Turner, T (1994) Paradox in practice. *Nursing Times*, **90**(21): 18.
UKCC (1986) *Project 2000: A New Preparation for Practice*. London: UKCC.

UKCC (1992a) *Code of Professional Conduct*. London: UKCC.
UKCC (1992b) *Standards for Incorporation into Contracts for Hospital and Community Health Care Services*, Registrar's letter 37/1992. London: UKCC.
Wright, S (1990) *Building and Using a Model of Nursing* (2nd edn.). London: Edward Arnold.

CHAPTER 3
Professionalism and Professional Qualifications
Betty Kershaw

> The debate about professionalism in nursing has never been out of the news for long. This chapter focuses on this debate from the ethical angle.
> A detailed analysis of what characterises a professional nurse is argued in a very immediate way, relating to practical issues and problems. Areas of practice are highlighted that may not always appear to be obviously questionable but which the author encourages every reader to think about.
> The blueprint of nursing as 'companionship' forms the conclusion to this chapter, a conclusion which must surely be taken seriously in today's debate about professionalism and professional qualifications.

Each registered nurse, midwife and health visitor shall act, at all times, in such a manner as to justify public trust and confidence, to uphold and enhance the good standing and reputation of the profession, to serve the interests of society, and above all to safeguard the interests of individual patients and clients.
(UKCC Code of Professional Conduct 1983)

Since the first Code of Professional Conduct was published, there has been one revision (1984) and one complete rewrite (1992). The choice to head this chapter with a quotation from the first edition was deliberate, simply because it marked the start of such an approach. Although nurses first entered the professional register in 1919 (and their midwife colleagues at the earlier date of 1902/3), this was the first attempt to bring our common professional responsibilities under one shared goal that clearly encompassed the accountability to and for patients and their care. The Nurses, Midwives and Health Visitors Act 1979 prompted the 1983 Code, its revision and the publication, in 1992, of the UKCC's *Scope of Professional Practice*. In this document, the accountability of the nurse for professional practice is further emphasised. However, we will initially consider the first Code of Professional Conduct.

The United Kingdom Central Council (UKCC) is charged by the above legislation to 'establish and improve the standards of training and professional conduct for nurses, midwives and health visitors' and to provide 'advice for nurses, midwives and health visitors on standards of professional conduct'. These statements are very closely integrated with nursing's ethical framework for practice and provide very clear evidence of its emergence as a profession, responsible and accountable for its own behaviour. It is no coincidence (Salvage 1985) that the UKCC, and the National Boards for England, Scotland, Wales and Northern Ireland, which support its activities and actions, were for the first time composed primarily of nurses rather than the medical professionals who played a leading role in monitoring the public (and institutional) accountability of the profession until that time. We have now (1993) moved even further towards corporate professional responsibility, in that the Council of the UKCC is two-thirds directly elected and only one-third nominated by either the Secretary of State or the four National Boards. The election is seen by some as being even more representative of the profession in that the voters use proportional representation. Some of the Council's power seems to be lost, however, when one realises that fewer than 20 per cent of eligible nurses, midwives and health visitors bothered to vote in the UKCC Council elections.

In order to move to explore further the issue of professional qualifications and ethical behaviour, it is necessary to go into the literature that explores the growth of nursing as a profession. Much of that literature grew out of the work of American colleagues in the 1940s, 1950s and 1960s. Their interpretative summaries are familiar to many nurses who have undertaken degree and diploma studies. One such summary comes from Holle and Blatchley (1982), who see professionals as those who:

> practice a full-time vocation that is the individual's source of income,
> have had an advanced education,
> have made a commitment to a particular calling,
> are identified by membership in a formalized organization,
> have a service orientation to humanity,
> have expertise that permits an autonomy circumscribed only by an associated responsibility and code of ethics.

Vocation

Professionals 'practice a full-time vocation that is the individual's source of income', according to Holle and Blatchley (1982). Salvage (1985) equates vocation with the concepts of religious service (nuns), idealism and 'angels'. She mentions such terms as self-sacrifice and service as being associated with 'ideal' nurses but counsels against ignoring the good things about a vocation, such as caring, compassion and patience. White (1985) explores vocationalism within the concept of the 'doctor's handmaiden', incorporating many of the criticisms that Salvage quotes above. White blames the reinforcement of that idea on the nurse education system, which indoctrinated that role both within the school of nursing and on the wards.

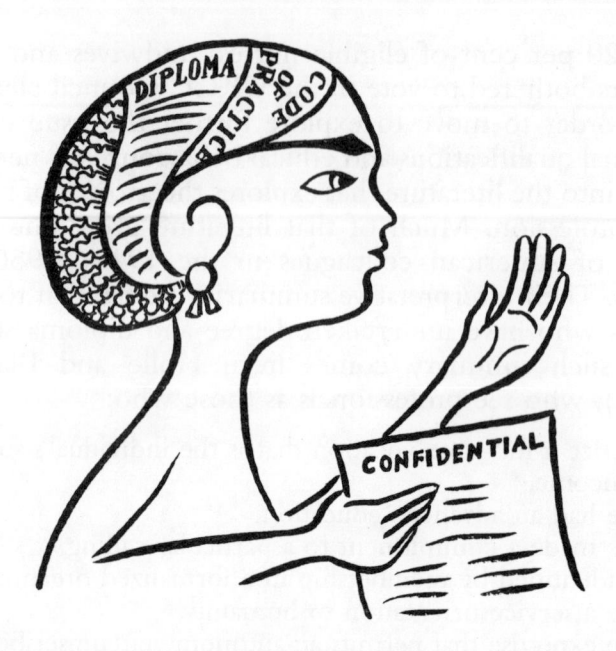

The preparation of nurses prior to Project 2000 (UKCC 1986) was primarily institutionalised, with ward sisters trained under the apprentice-type system introduced by Florence Nightingale in the 19th century. Salvage also saw training as having 'more to do with the needs of the medical profession than the notion that caring was a skill which should be developed'.

Dolan (1993) documents the changes in the profession that Project 2000 courses bring. We should now be seeing the move away from the service orientation detailed by White and Salvage towards something of which we can be proud, as it concentrates on developing the good qualities of caring. These have much to do with 'reasonableness, honesty, decency, honour and integrity' (Middleton 1983). However, the idea of vocation should be combined with education so that both can contribute to a profession facing the future.

The UKCC Code of Professional Conduct is about

accepting responsibility for the vocation of caring. Caring involves all the above qualities, but it is very difficult to be accountable for them through such approaches as formal audit, especially when these audits relate so often to quantity, performance indicators and numbers. Being accountable for caring must be encouraged through innovations that enhance the role of the nurse at delivery level and help the acceptance of accountability through responsibility and the quality of service delivery.

The early 1970s saw the introduction in the UK of the nursing process — the systematic approach to nursing care that revolves around the cycle or spiral of assessment, care planning, care delivery, evaluation and reassessment. At each stage, the nurse is required to document actions, decisions and goals for the next stage that are agreed with the patient and family or friends. Accountability is clearly there and is documented at every stage. Initially, nurses tended to base their assessments on the more familiar medical model, but by the time Surman was writing (1989), she noted the caring role of the nurse documented within the records. Whereas medical notes concentrated on, for example, constipation, reduction in blood pressure or dieting as directed, it was the nurse who concentrated on recording the giving of information to change eating habits, who talked to the patient about what he or she liked, basing dietary change upon these food and drink items, and explained to the patient and family how quality of life (and life expectancy) would improve with this new approach.

Before nurses can carry out any care, one needs to consider the issue of registration. Although nurses are all now designated Registered Nurse (RN) with the specific area of competence (care of the child, for example) identified in supporting information, they are so often still seen as 'interchangeable' (Salvage 1985; Dolan 1993), despite the fact that the Department of Health, when discussing health care assistants or support workers, specifically recommends that they are trained for their area of work and receive an additional course if they move placements or workplace. The UKCC (1990) also recommends similar updates for nurses moving from one area to another or returning to practice after a break. If students following Project 2000 courses are competent in the area of care for which they study at branch level, and must complete a 12-month programme of study and experience if they wish to change fields, one of the first ethical questions one must ask is whether or not, for example, general nurses should even be caring for children. Yet so often they are. Or should an RMN be working with clients who have learning difficulties? If a nurse is not competent, can he or she really provide care?

Having recognised competence to plan care, problems arise in the very nature of assessment. Nursing assessment must be comprehensive (Wright 1989), identifying patient needs within the psychological, social and physical domains of care. However, this in itself brings conflict. Increasingly, the political climate in which care is given is constrained through costs. How useful, helpful, or even ethical is it to identify a need which cannot be met? Examples abound:

- The elderly patient who has had a stroke and who needs a chair-lift so that he can continue to live at home: how many social service departments will support the application? And even if they do, how long will it take until the chair-lift is installed at home? Is it ethical for a registered nurse (general) to raise such expectations?

- The young man with long-term alcohol problems who has been assessed as needing community support: how can the registered nurse (mental health) raise his hopes at a time when services are being reduced? All nurses qualified in the area of disability care must be concerned about such news items as carried by *The Guardian* on March 4th 1993, which reported on victimisation and bullying of those residents living alone in small homes. How useful, practical, or ethical is it to encourage (indeed at times, virtually enforce) community care when we know that supportive services are not available?

The ethical issues abound, as do the pressures on nurses to function 'interchangeably'. The 1992 RCN Congress debated at length what nurses should do when they complain under the UKCC Code of Professional Conduct and no action is taken. The debate recognised the conflicts that managers have but also laid some blame at their door for insisting that nurses increasingly work outside their area of competence.

Professional Education

Holle and Blatchley (1982) see the second role in their definition of a professional as being '[one] who has had advanced education'. The UKCC Code of Professional Conduct (1992a) has consistently recognised that a registered nurse must maintain and improve his or her professional knowledge and competence. We have already seen how working in another area of care could be seen as unethical if it is outside a nurse's area of competence.

Is it ethical to care at all if nurses have not updated their knowledge or competence? *The Scope of Professional Practice* (UKCC 1992b) addresses this in depth, and all four National Boards have moved to assist nurses to do it. The National Board for Scotland began its work on diploma level practice-based courses as long ago as 1981. Under the chairmanship of Margaret Auld, the then chief nurse, this was a vision of the future that moved the profession on to diploma level studies (SHHD, 1981). The clinical nursing courses that were offered by individual hospitals were coordinated in the early 1970s by the Joint Board of Clinical Nursing Studies (JBCNS). The clinical courses developed by the JBCNS were incorporated into National Board courses in 1983, and in England are in the process of being incorporated into the English National Board framework and its Higher Award (ENB 1991). Currently, 27 colleges in England offer the programme; many more will be on-line in the near future. Scotland, as mentioned above, already has a well-established programme. Northern Ireland and Wales have similar opportunities. These courses, which lead on to degree level studies for those who want them, offer the opportunity to develop increased clinical competence based on sound knowledge.

As opportunities develop, how ethical is it not to follow such a programme while still maintaining competence within a professional remit? Nursing is increasingly becoming more technical; it is also demanding that practitioners develop skills of counselling, techniques of massage and reflexology; nurse prescribing is on the horizon, and the role of the nurse as a therapist is becoming a key to many innovations in practice and treatment. How ethical is it to practise in these areas of competence without updating and without having one's competence verified? The ENB Higher Award will allow nurses to develop this; at a lesser level so will the UKCC's PREPP (Post-registration Education and Practice Project) (1990) initiative. We owe this updating of competence to our patients and clients, as well as to those we work with and for.

Commitment

Holle and Blatchley's (1982) third area of professional recognition is that the individual 'has made a commitment to a particular calling' — in this case, the calling is obviously nursing and, more specifically, the special area in which one is competent and qualified.

The UKCC expects further preparation before nurses work within a new area of care. There can be no argument about this. No one expects a gynaecologist to cross theatres and replace hips, nor a paediatrician to do the geriatrician's clinic just because the latter is off sick. Neither would an industrial lawyer advise on a matrimonial dispute or a history teacher take the physics class. The devaluing of nurses' professional qualifications has gone on for many years, aided by those nurses who take over everyone else's roles and jobs once it is 5 pm on a Friday. When the physiotherapist is off, who does the physiotherapy? When the junior doctor is asleep, what does the night sister do? So often, nurses have rushed to take on the work of others, leading to the title 'Jack of all trades and master of none'. However, there is at long last some firm research evidence demonstrating that staff development, through the provision of post-qualification training, investment in employing qualified staff and developing effective methods of organising nursing care, pays 'dividends in the delivery of good quality and patient care' (Carr-Hill 1992). This report of the Centre for Health Economics at the University of York concentrates on quality of care within acute units. There is every reason to expect the findings to be similar when the study is repeated in any other nursing setting.

Cooper and Hornback (1973) recognised that nurses who were committed to caring for patients in particular settings or with special needs sought out staff development and in-service training that enabled them to care more efficiently and effectively. Wright (1989) documents at length how nursing practice was changed for the better when staff development was offered to nurses (and auxiliaries) who were committed to caring for the elderly and who saw further nursing knowledge and the development of new skills as being relevant to their needs. He records the improvement in the quality of care, in patient recovery rates and in staff stability; all this is evidence of a level of job satisfaction that one expects when nurses are working in the area of care that interests them, in which they hold their professional qualification and 'where they have made a commitment to a particular calling' (Holle and Blatchley 1982). Now that we have evidence to demonstrate that education and staff development improve care, is it ethical to continue to nurse without pursuing our own professional development?

There is a further point of relevance to this commitment, while we are considering specialisations within nursing. We have recognised that children should be cared for by children's nurses. Hawthorn's seminal research study, *Nurse – I want my Mummy*! was published in 1974 and has left no doubt in anyone's mind that such an approach is best for children, their families and the staff within the multidisciplinary team. Similarly, psychiatric patients need RMNs and, when living in the community, community psychiatric nurses. Those who have any contact with clients who have learning disabilities need no convincing of the value of their professional qualifications. The ethical issue of providing the best possible quality care is only achieved in this way.

But consider the RGN, who is expected to do everything, everywhere, every time and sometimes with public encouragement. In 1990, Reg Pyne, Director of Professional Conduct at the UKCC, wrote:

> I recall that for a significant period in the 1970's there regularly appeared in the national press . . . an advertisement placed by the Department of Health and Social Security aimed at encouraging young people to train as nurses. The words . . . urged those who saw and read it to see the . . . SRN (now RGN) as a passport to the world.

As Pyne reminds us, this is no longer accurate. However, it is certainly seen as a passport to being the general nurse who can work anywhere where adults — and indeed frequently people who have mental health or learning disability needs, and (of course) children — are cared for. The RGN qualification may not be a passport to the world, but so often it seems to mean that one can be moved at will. At a *Nursing Times* conference for ward sisters (April 2nd 1993), Roger Dyson, Professor in Health Management at the University of Keele, spoke with enthusiasm about a unit that operated as a surgical ward 10 months a year and a medical ward for the remaining 2 months — using the same nursing staff. He seemed to consider this an appropriate use of nurses, enabling them to provide high quality care. He was unable to assure his audience that the consultant surgeon became the consultant physician for two months as well. Like so many non-nurses, he devalues nursing skills and thus the care that nurses give.

We have to beware of such 'innovations' and ask ourselves where nurses would stand (within the UKCC Code of Professional Conduct 1992a) in relation to the following clauses, which demand that the nurse should:

- act always in such a manner as to promote and safeguard the interests of patients and clients;
- ensure that no action or omission on your part, or within your sphere of responsibility, is detrimental to the interests, condition or safety of patients and clients;
- maintain and improve your professional knowledge and competence;
- acknowledge any limitations in your knowledge and competence and decline any duties or responsibilities unless able to perform them in a safe and skilled manner.

A nurse who has made a commitment to a particular area of care will already be skilled in meeting the needs of that patient or client group. He or she will have built up expertise and a sound knowledge-base and will be well used to managing and delivering care. What ethical problems will confront the specialist practitioner in ophthalmic nursing who is reallocated, without opportunity to update and develop competence, to the paediatric unit, from theatre to care of the elderly or from male surgery to female neuromedicine? The suggestions are endless. The ethical point is not only that nurses are asked or expected to be interchangeable, but also that they have let themselves be so used. The ethical response to this must surely be 'no', more firmly put more often than in the past.

Professional Identification

Professionals are also 'identified by membership in a formalized organization' (Holle and Blatchley 1982). Nurses are already (through registration with their professional body, the UKCC) — and are increasingly becoming more so — involved in professional organisations that are rather more than trade unions. They offer the opportunity for networking and individual development and facilities to discuss and debate with nurses who share common interests. The Royal Colleges of Nursing and Midwives both have specialist interest groups and offer educational programmes that are available for their members who wish to update their knowledge-base for competence. The Royal Colleges have also been at the forefront of ethical debates. Ethics is invariably a major issue at the annual Congress of the RCN, being introduced into debates where even the most hardened politician would find it difficult to spot it at first. Some of the resolutions for the 1993 Congress (RCN 1993a) are immediately obviously ethical in origin:

That this meeting of the RCN Congress urges Council to campaign to make the process of rationing of health care more democratic.

That this meeting of the RCN Congress urges Council to lobby appropriate departments to establish a code of accountability for general managers working with the NHS and independent sector.

That this meeting of the RCN Congress urges Council to use its power to ensure that the professional skills of nurses are not diluted by re-profiling of the workforce.

That this meeting of the RCN Congress discuss the nurse's role in the management of a terminally ill patient in intractable pain, and the support necessary for nurses who disagree with prescribed medical interventions.

That this meeting of the RCN Congress requests Council to seek guidance from the UKCC regarding what nurses should do next when, having followed the Code of Professional Conduct, no action is taken by management.

Whistleblowing, euthanasia, replacing nurses by health care assistants or auxiliaries, the problems that arise when nurses, midwives and doctors are accountable as professionals for their ethical and professional behaviour but their managers are not, are issues that are of concern to all nurses. There are increasing conflicts when those practitioners at the 'coal face' are bound by the professional codes that guide their attitude and ethos to care, yet those who manage them are not bound by similar codes. The development of professional behaviour is instilled in professionals through their education and socialisation into the profession and is a key aspect of professional qualification. It is interesting to note that as the RCN debates the need for managers to have a code of conduct, there are calls for social workers to be bound by one, too.

The UKCC is also responsible for monitoring the professional registers. It provides a disciplinary framework for guaranteeing public assurance of the professional qualifications of nurses, midwives and health visitors, at which those professionals who are accused of misconduct are subject to a disciplinary hearing by a group of peer professionals with the same qualifications who bring to the enquiry their inside knowledge of the competence needed. The value of a professional qualification in maintaining the ethical standards of the professions is thus demonstrated yet again.

Service to Humanity

Professionals (Holle and Blatchley 1982) also have 'a service orientation to humanity'. The Code of Professional Conduct (1992a) also recognises responsibility to clients or patients but does not go as far as 'service to humanity', whose ethos is tied up with vocation. Salvage (1985) equates an idea of vocation with the image of nurses as 'angels'. The Cambridge Encyclopaedic Dictionary (1991) directly links Salvage with Holle and Blatchley by defining 'vocation' as:

> feeling that one is called (and qualified for) a certain kind of work, especially social or religious.

The editors of the Dictionary quote Florence Nightingale, 'Nursing is a vocation as well as a profession', to support their definition. The Dictionary recognises that one can now be educated for a vocation, especially by following courses validated by professional organisations, such as the National Boards for Nursing, Midwifery and Health Visiting; thus, the ideas of vocation and calling are no longer simplistic, with an air of 'too good to be true', but are now seen as necessary working models when combined with education.

It would appear, therefore, that nurses have a service commitment to humanity, which is often seen as a vocation. This service commitment necessarily brings responsibility, and, as there is no responsibility without accountability, this means for nurses accountability to the Code of Professional Conduct and the legislative requirements of practice and public protection.

Nowhere is this responsibility more challenged in the field of ethics than when one considers the issues of strikes (see Chapter 2 in *Conflicts of Interests* in this series). The RCN's constitution (1993b), Rule 12, clearly forbids strike action, but Rule 12 is increasingly challenged by members on the floor of Congress. This happened in 1993 under the item headed 'Industrial action': 'That this meeting of Congress discuss the current RCN position on industrial action'. The debate always makes it very obvious that service commitment to patients or clients is very strong among nurses but that they are becoming increasingly irritated by this ethical standard being taken for granted. Nurses have gone on strike in the UK. 1979 was the so-called 'winter of discontent', which saw nurses at the picket lines with other health care workers. Many found this disconcerting; others saw it as a way forward, while yet more nurses compromised their consciences by working to rule or only within their job descriptions. There is no doubt that this can be disruptive to patient care, but many nurses feel that it allows them to maintain their own ethical standards. It also allows them to feel 'better' than those who strike. This feeling is reported by Kalisch and Kalisch (1985) when describing nurses' action in the USA, where nurses do strike, though in small proportion (they cite 290 cases). It would appear that this is no more approved of by the nursing hierarchy in the USA than it is here.

But how does one equate personal and professional ethics with care, when standards of care are constantly being eroded by policies that are altering the skill mix and functions of nurses, are passing nursing activities to non-nurses and are reducing the quality of care that can be given to patients and clients? Kalisch and Kalisch (1985) saw the US strike action as being in part in defence of standards of care when contractual services of nursing were being reduced.

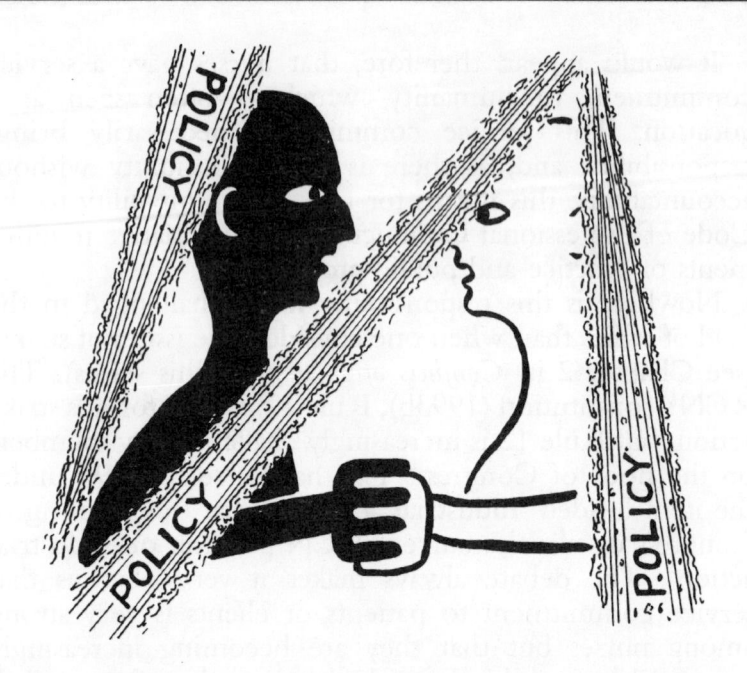

There is an alternative side to vocation that is personified in following voluntary organisations, for example VSO (Voluntary Services Overseas) or many of the groups serving Rumanian orphanages or Albanian psychiatric hospitals. This service orientation is often seen as truly vocational in that it is either non-paid or poorly paid. At its ultimate, it is apparent in those who join religious orders and become nuns or monks, who give their services free. (In reality they do earn salaries, but the salaries are paid to their house or order and not to the individual.) The services they have become involved in were (and are)

those which the public see as vocational and caring, such as teaching and nursing.

The numbers of nurses who are combining religious calling with professional activity are nominal in the UK. Salvage (1985) believes that the role they play diminishes the financial and professional work that people attribute to such jobs. The caring role has been rewarded with gratitude and respect, not least because many carers were to be found in hospitals for the elderly, the long-term mentally ill and mentally handicapped and the 'chronic sick'. Whitney (1988) recognises the part such nurses have played in giving care in these hospitals before the evolution of the NHS. Perhaps one reason for the spiralling costs of the NHS is the politicisation of nurses (and through them women) in their demands for equality and recognition. Kalisch and Kalisch (1985) see this as one of the demands of the nurses' strike in the USA.

If it is this factor that is contributing to costs and the diminishing money available for care, how do you, the reader, feel about the large pay awards that were given to nurses in the 1970s and 1980s? Does it trouble your ethical conscience to think that there is a direct relationship?

Autonomy

The final reason why Holle and Blatchley (1982) describe nursing as a profession is that nurses have 'expertise that permits an autonomy circumscribed only by an associated responsibility and code of ethics'. Professional autonomy is something that many nurses would like to have. (Chapter 4, describing midwifery practice, outlines probably the only area in which 'nurses' can be as autonomous as is possible.)

There are arguments for and against autonomy in nursing practice. Well-experienced and trained nurses need professional autonomy in order to care holistically for patients. They need autonomy to decide quickly and appropriately in cases of emergency. They need to have freedom from medical and bureaucratic interference in their decisions and freedom to decide how much information to give to patients and clients, or to colleagues. Such autonomy is only possible with responsibility that is set within the framework of a code of ethics.

Having professional autonomy is also dangerous. It can lead to overconfident decisions, which may have fatal consequences. The name of Beverley Allitt, the nurse who killed and injured a dozen babies, will remain on nurses' minds for a long time to come. It can be argued that she was sick and that this was the cause of her actions, but, sick or not, she practised as an enrolled nurse and, as such, was responsible for her actions.

The debate about the extended practice of nurses has been addressed by the UKCC in *The Scope of Professional Practice* (1992b). Since practice is constantly changing, registered nurses have to update their knowledge to maintain competence and the need to meet their PREP obligations. The documents point out, however, that to concentrate on 'activities' 'can detract from the importance of holistic nursing care'. Extension could lead to an isolation that may be detrimental to care. The increased autonomy that is offered by extension may not be welcome.

Nevertheless, nurses have autonomy in increasing fields of work. Nurse prescribing (Morris 1994) and Nursing Development Units (Jones 1994) are just two such areas. Community nurses and nurses in general practitioner practices also exercise a high degree of autonomy, as do school nurses and occupational health nurses. Their autonomy gives them a power that is necessary for practice, but this power has to be set within a clear framework of accountability.

Nursing constantly needs to find the equilibrium between autonomy and dependence. No freedom is absolute; moral, ethical and practical freedom is only possible when seen within the context of other people's lives, in particular those for whom nurses are responsible.

It is right that nurses should not be the doctors' handmaidens — equality is more helpful in the long run than inequality — but the idea of nursing as both vocation and job has also to be developed within a framework of cooperation with other health carers. Nursing has sought independence through its research. Perhaps it is becoming clearer now that research alone will not give nurses autonomy — if by that is meant independent professional status — but what will make nursing autonomous is clear responsibility and ethical thinking and acting.

Conclusion

The issue of ethical frameworks for practice is becoming more, rather than less, confused as the society we live and nurse in changes. The field of professional conflict and ethics is, therefore, likely to become more public as the stress in the health service rises. Carr-Hill (1992) reports on the value of qualified staff in giving care, but most of the ethical debates seem to arise from the standards of care expected, difficulties in meeting the quality nurses expect of themselves and a constant feeling of failure to maintain their own professional perspective.

RCN Congress debaters raise all these issues time and time again. We hear comments on skill mix analysis and about reports 'getting lost' when they demonstrate that more nurses are needed. We hear comments about standards not being met, and, therefore, being changed to meet a lower goal, and we hear of nurses being constantly subjected to stress because they cannot nurse to the standard they expect of themselves. There is no doubt that professional nurses are going to have to continue fighting to defend their ethical perspective for care. One way to do this successfully is to explore nursing's professional ethical framework, alongside those of other caring professions.

Campbell (1984), writing on professional care, recognises the personal perspective in our ethical behaviour and offers a philosophical framework for the caring professional that could become a model for ethical behaviour in the future. He debates professional care through vocation and raises the question of 'love', love for fellow human beings, compassion and caring. All these are hallmarks not just of nursing but also of the two other professions he addresses in his book: medicine and social work. Campbell was writing 10 years before caring in the community became official policy and certainly could not visualise the ways in which these three professions have to work together in the 1990s to deliver care. Neither could he have projected the rapid throughput scenario, nor the many multi-disciplinary team members who interface with patients and clients as they move from community to hospital, to home, to hospital (and home again).

Campbell's philosophy of caring 'companionship' fits well with the topical issues of the named nurse and primary nursing. He sees a patient's or client's interaction with health care professionals as a journey, in which the nurse, doctor or social worker assumes a partnership role. In referring this philosophy to nursing, he describes the nurse as 'the interpreter', as having 'sensitivity', as giving 'encouragement' and as being 'loyal', 'knowledgeable' and 'gentle'. He or she brings all these skills to the patient relationship and, because of the professionalism of the person, they form the basis of the ethical framework for care.

Using Campbell's philosophy of caring companionship, the carer, be he doctor, nurse or social worker, meets the patient, client and family for the first time and makes a professional contract to provide care and treatment through their hospital (or other) experience. The professional assists the person to adapt to the many changes experienced on that journey, encouraging, supporting, counselling, advising and treating, but remaining always aware that, as with all journeys, there will be an end. Thus, the professional comes professionally close but never becomes so involved that it is impossible to break the relationship, because the need for the relationship to end is part of the initial contract.

Campbell offers much for nurses. His ideas give strength to the arguments that the patient who is admitted to hospital for respite care, day-case surgery or rehabilitation should retain his or her community nurse as primary carer or (indeed) as 'named nurse'. He supports integrated care, offering all health professionals a framework from which to practise. His writings lend themselves to the present and future need to prepare and plan for discharge (and rehabilitation) at admission or even earlier. The companionship role can be especially compatible with the adaptation-based models of nursing and encourages nurses who aim to support patients through programmes of behaviour that concentrate on self-care philosophies. It also has something of relevance to course tutors and counsellors.

Campbell offers us a framework for professional ethical compatibility that could reduce conflict about who is responsible for what and all the other many power-based statements that often obstruct, albeit in a minimal way, the progress of patient care and treatment. Surely that is the goal of us all.

References

Cambridge Encyclopaedic Dictionary (1991) Cambridge: Cambridge University Press.
Campbell, AV (1984) *Moderated Love: A Theology of Professional Caring*. London: SPCK.
Carr-Hill, R (1992) *Skill Mix and the Effectiveness of Nursing Care*. Available from Centre for Health Economics, University of York, York YO1 5DD.
Cooper, SS and Hornback, HS (1973) *Continuing Nursing Education*. New York: McGraw Hill.
Dolan, B (1993) *Project 2000: Reflection and Celebration*. London: Scutari Press.
ENB (1991) *The Framework and the Higher Award*. London: ENB.
The Guardian (1993) Mental handicap people victimised when living in the community. News item, March 4th.
Hawthorne, P (1974) *Nurse — I Want my Mummy!* RCN Research Series. London: RCN.
Holle, M and Blatchley, MC (1982) *Introduction to Leadership and Management in Nursing*. Belmont, California: Wadsworth Health Sciences Division.
Jones, J (1994) White coats ousted from acute wards. *The Observer*, May 22nd.
Kalisch, B and Kalisch, P (1985) Nurses on strike — labour management conflict in our hospitals and the role of the press. In White, R, *Political Issues in Nursing: Past, Present and Future*. Chichester: John Wiley and Sons.
Middleton, D (1983) *Nursing 1*. Oxford: Blackwell Scientific Publications.
Morris, J (1994) Demonstration sites for nurse prescribing. *Nursing Times*, **90**(21): 31–2.
Nurses, Midwives and Health Visitors Act (1979). London: HMSO.
Pyne, R (1990) Introduction. In Kershaw, B, *Nursing Competence*. London: Edward Arnold.
RCN (1993a) *1993 Congress Agenda*. Available from the Royal

College of Nursing, 20 Cavendish Square, London W1M 0AB.
RCN (1993b) *RCN Constitution*. London: RCN.
Salvage, J (1985) *The Politics of Nursing*. London: Heinemann.
SHHD (1981) *A Report of the Working Party on Continuing Education and Professional Development for Nurses, Midwives and Health Visitors*. Available from the library, Scottish Home and Health Department, St Andrew's House, Regent Road, Edinburgh EH1 3DE.
Surman, L (1989) Theory into practice: some examples of the application of change strategies. In Wright, S, *Changing Nursing Practice*. Sevenoaks: Edward Arnold.
UKCC (1983, 1984 and 1992a) *Code of Professional Conduct for the Nurse, Midwife and Health Visitor*. London: UKCC.
UKCC (1986) *Project 2000: What it Is and What it Is Not*. London: UKCC.
UKCC (1990) *Post Registration Education and Practice Project (PREPP)*. London: UKCC.
UKCC (1992b) *The Scope of Professional Practice*. London: UKCC.
White, R (1985) *Political Issues in Nursing: Past, Present and Future*. Chichester: John Wiley and Sons.
Whitney, R (1988) *National Health Crisis*. London: Shepheard-Walwyn.
Wright, S (1989) *Changing Nursing Practice*. Sevenoaks: Edward Arnold.

CHAPTER 4
Independent Midwifery Practice
Caroline Flint

> Independent practice is a concept that is heard and tried again and again in nursing — but is it *really* possible in nursing? It has certainly been possible in midwifery for some time.
>
> The author, an independent midwife, makes a strong point that nursing and midwifery are two different professions with different aims. She writes from her own practice, highlighting ethical problems that are almost unknown in nursing. Thus, this chapter is different not only in that it is about midwifery rather than nursing, but also in style and content, offering a challenge to readers from a different point of view.

When approached by an editor asking me to write a chapter in a book about ethics concerning nurses and their patients, I am immediately thrown into an ethical dilemma as a midwife. I am a midwife who believes very strongly that midwifery and nursing are totally separate professions and that they should not be under the same legislation, nor have the same statutory body. Since 1979, much of my professional life has been devoted to trying to take midwives out of the legislation that surrounds nurses. So why am I writing a chapter about independent *midwifery* practice in a book about *nursing* ethics?

I am not writing about independent nursing practice because, as far as I can see at this moment, and I do not perceive any change in this in the foreseeable future, I do not believe that there can be truly independent nursing practice. There do not appear to be any areas of life that can be deemed as 'normal' and treated completely by nurses. Perhaps the care of the dying is a field in which nurses can practise independently, but as legislation does not exist for them to be able to prescribe the types of drug and the strengths of dose that many dying people require, nurses will, for the forseeable future, be controlled by, or working under the auspices of, the medical profession.

So, back to my dilemma. I am a midwife, committed to the separate nature of midwifery as a profession. I believe that midwifery and nursing have fundamentally different philosophical roots. I see nursing as rooted in caring, making sick people comfortable, relieving them — either of pain, anxiety or discomfort — acting as an advocate for them and complementing medical care. I see midwifery as a much tougher, perhaps less kind discipline.

The women a midwife deals with are healthy, often healthier than they have ever been in the whole of their life. They are assertive, they are aware that this is *their* pregnancy, *their* labour, *their* baby; that I am their employee, their servant, their assistant. I am there to support, to enable normal childbirth, to assure privacy, to advise — aware that my advice is not always taken.

The Ethical Principles Behind My Practice

Truth-telling

The fundamental premise of independent (and indeed all midwifery) practice is respect for a unique woman. This means that I should be completely truthful and honest with her. For some midwives who work within a busy hospital, truth-telling and honesty, two of the principal ethical values within any profession, can sometimes be difficult to deal with, mainly because of lack of time, but sometimes because of other pressures: from other midwives and from medical staff.

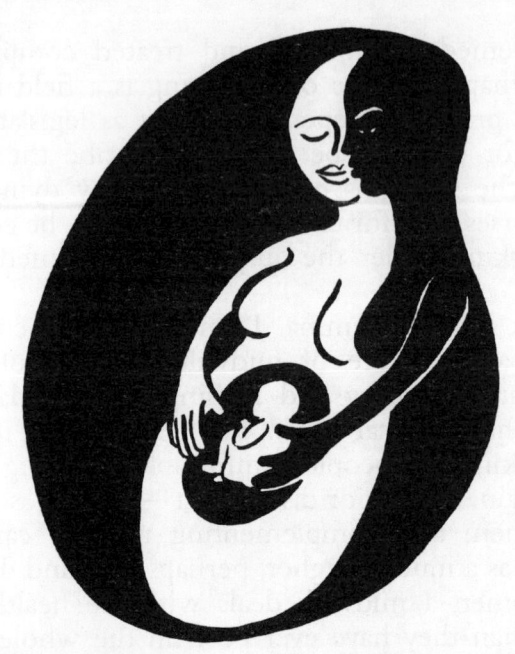

- I remember the ethical dilemma I felt when working in hospital when a consultant obstetrician turned to me and said in front of the woman she was talking with, 'We know that ultrasounds are harmless, don't we, Sister Flint? Mrs X is worried about having one.' What could I say? I had to be honest, but at the risk of incurring the wrath and displeasure of that particular obstetrician with whom I needed to work and whom I needed to influence and negotiate with. What I said was, 'I don't think we know conclusively that ultrasounds are safe, we haven't yet seen much harm done by them but there are several groups who feel that they haven't been tested enough to see what their long-term effects are, and in fact there have been one or two studies that have shown harmful effects of ultrasounds such as hearing problems, but there have not been enough conclusive research studies yet.' This small interaction soured our relationship for several months.

Empowerment

My aim is that women are empowered during the whole process of giving birth, that they are made stronger, more confident and grow from being a 'girl' to being a 'woman'. I do not expect to act as their advocate. I expect them to feel strong enough to tell me what they want of me and I hope that they will approve of my care. I hope that they will recommend my service to other women.

These feelings of being the 'employee' of women are obviously highlighted by being in independent practice and being directly employed by women, but they are relevant to all midwives. Those midwives working within the NHS (as most of them are) are employed by the state — which in essence means the people who are receiving the maternity services. Maybe this feeling of providing a service for healthy people has been the factor that has made maternity services much more 'consumer' dominated than other areas of health and ill-health provision.

Independent midwifery is concerned with a discrete episode of health in which a midwife can provide total care for a woman and her newborn baby. A woman can engage me as a practising independent midwife early in her pregnancy. I can provide her with checks throughout her pregnancy; I can order blood tests from a private laboratory at which I have an account; I can refer my client for an ultrasound scan at a private hospital where my practice has an account.

When a woman goes into labour, she calls my practice and either I or my practice partner responds to her call. We will go to her home and assess the situation, and if the labour progresses normally, we will usually stay in her home. We can prescribe and carry pethidine (intramuscular analgesic), Entonox (inhalational analgesic) and syntometrine (for hastening labour), but we rarely use these drugs. After the baby and the placenta are born, we can repair any perineal damage and also check the baby. So far, midwives cannot check the baby's heart sounds, so we refer the mother and her baby to their GP, who usually comes to check the baby within a few days of birth.

Health advice

The midwife visits and provides health advice for the mother and baby for the subsequent 28 days of the life of this new family. Immediately after the birth, we usually help a woman to the bath and help her to wash herself clear of blood from the birth. During the next few days, we will bath the baby and show the mother how to do this; often we change the baby's nappy or weigh the baby. We take blood from the baby for the phenylketonuria test or from the mother to check on her haemoglobin levels. We usually carry out physical checks on both mother and baby for at least 10 days after the birth, and usually visit mother and baby for four weeks following the baby's birth.

Choice

Over the period of a pregnancy, we get to know women very well, and sometimes we give the woman research evidence that may perhaps mean that she should change her decision from having her baby at home to delivery in hospital; likewise, during a homebirth, we may advise transfer to hospital. It is up to the woman whether or not she takes our advice, and this in itself can be very disturbing and can provide a very strong ethical dilemma. However, the Midwife's Code of Practice (UKCC 1991) is clear and in this instance is very helpful:

4.2 In a situation where a midwife considers that home confinement is inappropriate and the mother refuses to take the advice of the midwife to receive care in a maternity unit the midwife must continue to give care and consult her supervisor of midwives, making an appropriate record.

4.3 In some instances a midwife may require medical assistance for a mother booked for a home confinement but the mother or her partner may refuse to have the registered medical practitioner in attendance. If this situation arises the midwife must continue the care of the mother and consult as soon as possible with her supervisor of midwives, making an appropriate record.

A midwife can be in a very difficult position, for instance when a woman is bleeding, the midwife wants to give an injection of syntometrine but the woman says very firmly, 'No, I do not want it.' Many people believe that if a midwife has a very good relationship with a woman, the latter will trust and always comply with the midwife's advice. In my experience, this is not so. The type of relationship that one has with women enables them to make their own decisions very strongly. Undoubtedly, most women will take the advice of a midwife they trust, but some women feel so strongly and so passionately about specific aspects of their care that, despite all good advice and well-documented research being made available to them, they still are unable to comply with the midwife's suggestion. The Midwife's Code of Practice is very supportive here and exemplifies respect for the individual person.

Being self-employed

As an independent midwife, I am self-employed, which means I am responsible for my own income. It means that I have no pension and no sick pay unless I arrange these for myself. It means taking on a greater degree of responsibility for my own wellbeing than is experienced by people who are employed. It means that I need to gain a certain degree of business acumen. I must charge a realistic amount so that I cover the costs of the provision of the service, but also I must not charge so much that no-one will book my practice, perceiving it as too expensive.

A great ethical dilemma concerns those women who want to use our practice but cannot afford us. We practise in London, so we are able to send women who cannot afford us to independent midwives who charge less than we do; we help women to get the service they are wanting from their local NHS services; we can have an 'easy' payments scheme spread over a period of years but this can be uneconomic; we take credit card payments, but they are subject to certain charges. All these options cost us in either time or money. We are negotiating with a finance company to prepare a package that we could offer to women, which would then enable us to be paid immediately and enable the parents to pay over a period of time. If people have private health insurance, they are not covered for normal births, so this does not help at all.

Financial dilemmas

For many midwives working in private/independent practice, finance is a huge dilemma. Most midwives working in independent practice do not really want to be in private practice and do not espouse the values of private medicine; they actually want to care for women in the best way they know. They want to provide continuity of carer; they want to support women and enable them to give birth in the way and in the place that they want to. The women they look after do not have very much money and are often exceedingly poor. Many of these midwives (and I have been interested to meet midwives working in this way all over the world) provide their care for very low fees and sometimes for nothing at all. The service these midwives give is wonderful and the way they practise is exemplary; they are working at the deepest human level of self-sacrifice and dedication.

But there is another ethical dilemma about finance: the mortgage has to be paid, food has to be bought, the car has to be maintained — all of this costs money. All too often, midwives go out of practice, being unable to continue to work in the way that they want, because they just cannot afford to work like that any longer. Some midwifery practices are trying to contract into the NHS for their services to be purchased by individual health services.

As an independent midwifery practice, we must buy all our own equipment, disposables, drugs, bags, bleepers, portable phones, cars, education material, books, syringes, needles, suture materials, sanitary towels, incopads, oxygen, Entonox and resuscitation equipment. We must provide ourselves with an office, telephone, accountant, solicitor, financial adviser, printer, graphic designer, secretary and locum if we go away. All the costs of our business/practice are tax deductible, but this requires a certain discipline because every gallon of petrol we buy, every pen, typewriter ribbon, ream of paper and box of sanitary towels must be recorded and the invoice kept; with a business involving the purchase of 5000 incopads per year alone, the documentation of purchases has to be a daily task — fine at slack times, a nightmare at busy ones.

The Choice of an Independent Midwife

Why do women choose to go to an independent midwife? Why do they choose to pay for a service that in many ways is almost exactly the same as the service provided by the NHS free of charge? The reason has been stated by women for years:

> She would like, if it were possible, to have someone around during her labour who had given her some antenatal care.
> (Micklethwaite et al 1978)

> It has been suggested to us that women should have the same midwife to attend them in labour as in the antenatal period. We consider this continuity of care to be an ideal aim and it may be possible in some circumstances.
> (Royal College of Obstetricians and Gynaecologists 1982)

> Mothers would like antenatal, delivery and postnatal care to be provided, as far as possible, by the same people. Again and again, letters expressed the anxiety that arises when seeing a different doctor at each visit to the antenatal clinic, and being delivered by total strangers — sometimes two different shifts of total strangers if a woman had a long labour.
> (Parents Magazine 1983)

> Good communications between parents and the medical staff were helped where women saw the same doctor and midwife regularly — most mothers saw different people at almost every antenatal visit and were delivered by total strangers. While full of praise for the care they received, many women wished they could have had more continuity of care through pregnancy and beyond.
> (Parents Magazine 1986)

> There is a strong desire among women for the provision of continuity of care and carer throughout pregnancy and childbirth ... the majority of them regard midwives as the group best placed and equipped to provide this.
> (Health Committee 1992)

> The evidence we have received suggests that the importance of continuity of care needs underlining very heavily for the professions who are involved in delivering the maternity services of the NHS. Many still demonstrate an insufficient

awareness of its prominence among the criteria which women use to judge the quality of the care they have received. Nor have they yet done nearly enough to respond in practical terms to the call by women to be involved as full partners in the decisions made about their care.
(Health Committee 1992)

When a woman is having a baby, nothing can replace the support of a known and trusted professional. Many women described to the Group the reassurance of seeing a familiar face at critical points, when they were anxious or when complications arose, but especially when they went into labour. They described the importance of being able to develop a relationship of trust, with 'my midwife' or 'my doctor', someone who is familiar with their antenatal history and their plans for the birth.
(Department of Health 1993)

I believe the most important is continuity of carer. The review team were haunted by the phrase we heard so often when talking to mothers: 'All I wanted was a familiar face'. This is, after all, a reasonable request. We should not subject women to having to relate to 30 or 40 professionals during their pregnancy, birth and immediate postnatal period.
(Cumberlege 1994)

The Association of Radical Midwives (1986) and the Royal College of Midwives (1987) both advocate that midwives should work in small teams and take responsibility for providing continuity of care for a specific group of women that they are able to get to know. Despite this, there has been a marked resistance by the midwifery profession to consider seriously the desire of women for continuity of care, this resistance being marked by the actual changing of the concept of 'continuity of care' into 'not continuity of care' by the same midwife or midwives throughout pregnancy, labour and the puerperium. The concept of 'continuity of care' means that every member of the obstetric team says the same thing and holds the same philosophy and that protocols and procedures are drawn up to this end:

> I am anxious that there should be real change — not just window-dressing. I have seen some excellent ideas fade as their terminology became diluted. A good example is 'domino' midwifery care. This initially meant that a community midwife should care for the mother in her home and then accompany her into hospital to deliver the baby, but it has been changed to mean simply a short stay in hospital. Similiarly 'holding own notes' has now shrunk to mean holding your own birthplan, and 'continuity of carer' to mean 'continuity of care' — which is something completely different.
>
> (Cumberlege 1994)

To overcome this concept, many midwives who are aware of what women want now talk about 'continuity of carer' rather than 'continuity of care'.

Despite the evidence that what women want and are asking the midwifery profession for is to be able to form a relationship with the person who will be with them during labour, it is still possible to hear midwives saying, 'I don't think mothers really mind who looks after them in labour as long as they are kind'. This mentality produces the situation in which a woman decides to have her baby at home or have a 'domino' delivery and then, when she approaches the community midwives to arrange it, she is told that when it comes to delivery she may have any one of 16 midwives to look after her during labour. She will have a chance to 'meet' the midwife at a tea party or coffee morning. This is so unsatisfactory and such a long way from what they actually want that some women will go to great lengths to avoid it, even paying £2000 or more to engage an independent midwife and financially overstretching themselves.

The Model of Woman-based Care

What do midwives working independently offer to women that is special? Perhaps their care should become the model on which all maternity care should be based. Going through step by step what a woman receives from an independent midwife from booking until discharge begins to show the reason why women choose this type of care.

The initial contact

The first contact a woman and independent midwife will have with each other is over the telephone, the woman asking the independent midwife about her services and her charges. Most independent midwives tell women about their right to have a baby at home with a community midwife, but women have usually explored that avenue and have either felt intimidated when told that home confinements 'aren't done in this district', have been misinformed that 'there are no GPs who do home deliveries and therefore we can't do them' or have been told of the 'any one of 16 midwives' who may care for them in labour.

The dilemma that an independent midwife has to explore, especially when her practice charges more than other independent midwives, is that of giving a woman choice. Many women do not know that they can have private obstetric care from an obstetrician who will provide continuity of care and will be with them during labour in a private hospital. If they are in a position to pay for independent midwifery, they need to be told about private obstetricians. They also need to be told about other midwives who provide the same service, often more cheaply. They need to be told about all the choices available to them even if it means that they actually do not end up with the midwife who is giving them all this information.

It is just another version of telling the truth and being open and honest with women and enabling them to have the freedom to make the choice that is best for them.

The first consultation

If the woman is interested in going ahead, she will make a date for a first consultation. This is an opportunity for the midwife and client to get to know each other, to look each other over and decide whether they are right for each other, and is an opportunity to discuss and negotiate fees, services, venues and all the other aspects of her care over which a woman wants to have control.

The first meeting will probably take place in the evening or at the weekend at the woman's house so that her partner can take part. This is the first principle upon which independent practice is based: the time when the consultation takes place is a time that is convenient for the woman and her partner. The consultation will take place in the woman's home; the midwife will stand outside the door and ring the bell: she is the stranger, the visitor. The woman will open the door and greet her, will show her a seat to sit on, will offer her a cup of tea (or not!). The woman is in control: it is her place, she is calling the tune. The immediate start of the relationship is based upon the woman deciding whom she will have to attend her and the type of care she chooses to have.

The first consultation usually begins with social chitchat: 'What a lovely view you have' or 'It is nice and cosy in here, isn't it?' The essence of normality, everyday affairs and interests pervades the air. This is a home, it is where somebody lives, it is normal and usual and mundane — nothing dramatic, pathological or ill is here.

Once the social small talk has been gone through, it is also likely to break through over and over again during the course of the consultation. The midwife will start to take a booking history, asking about the woman and her partner's medical histories, their families' health, the way her mother had babies, why they have decided on having a home birth and other relevant questions, but during the session threads will be drawn together: 'Oh your parents live in Marbella, do they? I went on holiday there when I was 15. Is the fish bar still on the front where you could get the most delicious . . .', 'You originally came from Leeds, did you? My sister lives there'. Both the parties are learning about each other, the midwife giving as well as receiving information; she begins to be known as well as getting to know.

The midwife will examine the woman physically, take her blood pressure, examine her hands and feet in order to assess her bone structure, examine her breasts for lumps and bumps, palpate her abdomen and examine her ankles for œdema. All this will be done in the woman's bedroom with the curtains drawn — private, familiar and normal, a place where the woman is used to being undressed, which smells like her place, looks like her place, is her place.

The midwife will test the woman's urine. The client's specimen will be produced in her own lavatory with the door shut — private and familiar.

Ongoing care

When the notes are completed, the midwife will make a copy of whatever is relevant for her information and will leave the notes with the woman and her partner; there are parts of it which they will be expected to fill in. The notes are the diary of a pregnancy, labour and puerperium, written by a midwife, a mother-to-be and a father-to-be. The notes are a shared record and kept in the woman's possession. After the care is finished and the diary is no longer kept, the midwife retains the original of the notes but gives the couple a photocopy for future reference and pleasure: 'Oh I'd forgotten that I felt so exhausted at the beginning of that pregnancy, and look, we had a row about the baby's names all through June and July of that year — whether it was going to be Jake or Jolyon and then it turned out to be Sarah!' All this serves to retain the woman's control over her pregnancy and what happens to her. It is her pregnancy, her labour, her post-natal period, her baby and her notes — her responsibility all the way through.

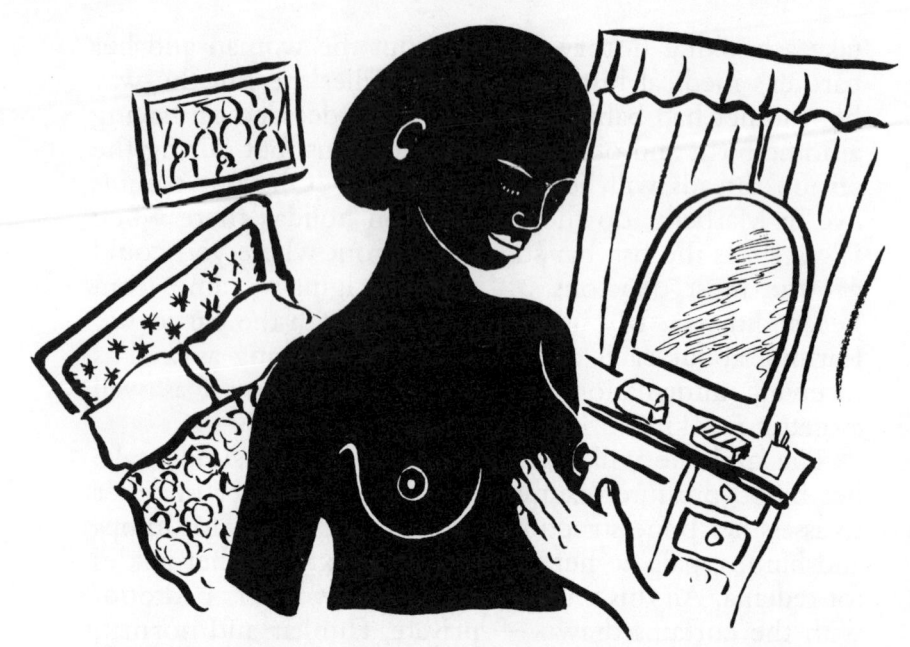

Throughout the pregnancy, antenatal consultations usually take place in the woman's home, but sometimes in the midwife's home or consulting rooms, a normal-looking environment that displays aspects of the midwife's personality — her books, her photos, the pictures she has on her wall, some of her son's toys lying around the floor. These are all indications of normality and 'everydayness'. The midwife looks normal and everyday; she wears the same sort of clothes as her clients wear; she obviously has the same sort of needs and problems that her clients have. She is another woman, a potential friend and ally, but it is the woman who is in charge, who is calling the tune and who is taking responsibility.

Motherhood

If we look at the nature of parenting, we can understand more easily the necessity for the couple, and especially the woman, to take control and responsibility for all the events surrounding the birth of her child. A mother in our society is valued only by her child; our society sees motherhood as an unpaid task of little significance, the 'real' work being done by merchant bankers in the City or by executives in smart suits who sit in first-class carriages on trains and talk to each other on their portable telephones. The woman toiling over her child's needs for food, exercise and play, to be kept clean, entertained, read to, played with, taught the basic fundamentals of life — all this is seen by society as by-the-by, not important and on the fringes of real existence. Consequently, when the woman goes out, if she tries to travel on public transport it is almost impossible to manage a pushchair, bag and baby without help. Shops are designed for babies to be somewhere else, restaurants are not a place where babies or small children are welcomed, museums have 'No pushchairs' notices and pubs are barred to small children. And as if this were not enough, most couples are financially more stretched than at any other time in the whole of their lives. The mother at home with her baby can feel totally isolated from the rest of society.

A mother has a job that is undervalued, where there are no markers or measures of success: no-one knocks on her door and says, 'Mrs Robinson, here is a bunch of flowers because everyone in the street thinks you are the best mother of all time.' No-one gives her a certificate for being a good mother; rather the opposite usually happens: 'My goodness, she isn't feeding again is she? You do spoil her'; 'Your Mary cries a lot, doesn't she?'; 'Your sister's children don't meddle with the ornaments as much as your Bobbie does.'

The mother who is denigrated and put down has to rely entirely on her own inner resources and any fragile peer support she can muster. But to her child, everything is different: the mother is a goddess, she knows everything, she controls everything, she is the source of all nourishment, all self-esteem, all fun and all pleasure — a deity, a wonder woman, more lovely, more clever, more exciting and more endearing than any other human being in the world. For a woman to take on that role, she needs to have huge self-confidence and vigour and a deep well of self-esteem, and most women know that the way in which they give birth will have a significant effect on how they feel about themselves.

In order to stay in control of the situation and to retain power and control over the birth process, the woman chooses to have her baby in her own surroundings, accompanied by those people she chooses to have with her and attended by a professional who is a visitor to her house and, therefore, in a subordinate position. The professional's concept of labour is that it is a normal life event. Women's bodies work, and the baby will come out healthily, given time. The midwife only needs to support and trust the woman, and the woman herself will know what to do and how to be. Obviously, that professional will detect any abnormalities if they crop up and will respond to them, but on the whole she does not expect them to occur — why should they? This is a healthy woman, is it not? Birth works, does it not? In her experience, birth is a normal event that works well, and women are in control of it.

When a woman has had this sort of encouragement throughout her labour, when she has laboured within an ethos that believes she **can** do it, when she has been surrounded by encouraging and congratulatory voices throughout her labour, when she has given birth and the assembled company has revolved around her — her needs, her desires, her brilliance at being a labouring mother, a birthing mother, a breast-feeding mother — then the world has stopped turning in deference to her amazing qualities as a mother. She grows in powerfulness and she grows rapidly into a mother — not just any old mother, but a brilliant mother, an exceptional mother, a mother recognised by others as brilliant. What better start in life as a mother can this feeling of powerfulness bring?

Oakley (1974–79) in her study 'Transition to motherhood' suggests that 'A woman who feels "master" of her own life is more likely to feel basically optimistic in the face of threatening change: she is able to visualize recovery from loss and the restructuring of identity and reward this entails.' In *Women Confined* (1984), Oakley also suggests that 'the medicalization of reproduction has changed the subjective experience of reproduction altogether, making dependence on others instead of dependence on self a condition of the achievement of motherhood.'

Paying for a Type of Service

Those women who are aware that in order to escape from having to be dependent on others they must pay someone to come to their house and deliver them there are the ones who choose to engage an independent midwife.

When the woman approaches labour, she will keep in touch with the midwife whom she knows really well by now. If she is worried that her membranes might have ruptured, she will inform the midwife, who will come and examine her. If she thinks that labour may have started, she will inform the midwife, who will come and assess what is going on, at all times. Twenty-four hours a day, seven days a week, she has access to a sympathetic and knowledgeable practitioner at the other end of a telephone, whom she knows and who knows her — a huge advantage for any pregnant woman.

When mutually agreed, the midwife will come to the woman's house and stay with her throughout her labour, although staying with her can mean many things. It does not usually mean staying glued to her side. It can mean the midwife sitting in front of the television or reading the newspaper in one room while the woman labours in another room with her partner. It can mean the midwife sleeping comfortably on the sofa while the woman relaxes in the bath. It can mean the midwife brewing up pots of herb tea or cooking slices of toast for the assembled company. It can mean the midwife massaging the woman's back or pouring water on her while she is in the bath.

Each woman is unique. Her needs are different from those of any other woman in the world, and she relaxes in the comforting knowledge that this midwife will recognise this. She will not be told, 'We shall rupture your membranes now because you are 4 centimetres dilated', or 'Most women enjoy going into the jacuzzi at this stage.' She knows that this labour is hers and will be treated as hers, almost as if she is the first woman ever to give birth — as indeed she is: the first woman to give birth in precisely *this* way.

The midwife will make sure that the fetal heart is regular and strong, that the woman remains well and that her bladder remains emptied. She will be watching in case any deviation occurs but will expect the labour to continue to a normal outcome. She will trust the woman's body to progress in labour and to give birth to a healthy baby. She has seen this before; she expects it to happen normally; she *knows* that it works.

The midwife sees it as the woman's right to have the sort of birth she wants and to be able to labour unfettered by doctrines or policies, but having with her a professional who respects the process and who respects the woman. It is the midwife's responsibility to enable the woman to tune into her deeper instincts and to give birth in the way that she wishes to.

After the baby is born, the pace is set by the woman. She may just want to curl up and opt out for a few minutes — half an hour, an hour — or she may be full of vigour and power, ecstatic and enthusiastic, putting the baby to the breast, exclaiming over the baby, thanking everyone, discussing why certain things happened and how certain things felt. She may be starving with hunger or feeling nauseated. Whatever she feels, she is secure in the knowledge that everyone is there for her and her alone, and they will cater for all her needs — she is Queen for the day, she is still calling the tune and the world revolves around her. Her baby is bathed, or cuddled, or lies in the big bath with her or with its father, or suckles or lies and looks around. What is done has no pattern, what is done is what needs to be done here for this mother and this baby. 'Usual practice' or 'our routine' do not have a place here; this situation is unique, a one-off occasion.

After the Birth

Once the birth is over, what happens about the developing of this woman into a mother? Each day, sometimes twice, sometimes three times, the midwife will visit, check, encourage, help and teach, but will always ask permission to touch the baby, because the baby belongs to the woman and the woman is in charge of the baby; the midwife is always the visitor. She will always encourage, support and compliment. The baby will be cared for in its own home, and the mother will learn to bath her in this home, change his nappy on this table or sitting in this chair, feed her sitting in this armchair, exercise on this mat — everything is geared to this house and how it is. Motherhood starts off in the woman's own environment. She learns expertise in a secure place where she is in charge. The midwife, a skilled practitioner, is the visitor, albeit by now a loved and familiar one. But the woman calls the tune all the way through.

The postnatal care goes on regularly daily until the baby is 10 days old. Then the visits begin to tail off: four days gap, then six days and so on until the baby has reached four weeks. The midwife says, 'I must now discharge you officially, but I'll come back in two weeks with the photocopy of your notes'. She is a helping hand through those first difficult six weeks, a time of huge change, tiredness and learning to understand this small person who has no concept of day or night but just feed time and then another feed time. The midwife is a friend and supporter throughout this unique experience.

The Midwife

Learning from practice

Those, then, are the benefits for the woman of independent midwifery practice. But what of the midwife herself? What benefits does she perceive from practising in this way? It has to be said that for most midwives practising independently, the benefits are being able to practise the full role of the midwife: caring for a woman from early in pregnancy until 28 days after delivery. She is able to benefit from the satisfaction of providing continuity of care, being able really to get to know the couple, really enter into the whole spirit of the labour and that family. As people in their infinite variety are fascinating, the midwife will feel privileged to be part of a unique and intimate experience. She will know that she will be for ever engraved on that couple's hearts, the 'our lovely midwife who said . . .', or 'Do you remember when Mary said, "Good heavens and I've only just started drinking this coffee and now it's nearly here".'

The midwife is also aware of learning very rapidly — being with a woman all the way through her pregnancy, labour and puerperium enables a midwife to learn very thoroughly. This experience enhances learning opportunities because the midwife can hear what the woman is saying and thus gain a huge amount of knowledge from the woman herself.

Responsibility

Another factor that enhances the satisfaction of independent midwives is that of being self-employed and having their own equipment. Not for them is the sonicaid in which the battery has gone flat — they are responsible for charging their own batteries. Not for them is the frustration of not being able to find a thermometer, because it is the midwife herself who supplies it. It is her responsibility and hers alone to equip herself satisfactorily. She buys for herself those pieces of equipment that *she* likes to use.

Independence

The other joy of practising independently is when working with a partner (as many independent midwives do) and the joy of seeing a different perspective through someone else's eyes. The support and encouragement from another midwife, the giggles and the fun, the anxieties and the worries, all shared, all enjoyed or despaired of together — twice the pleasure, half the agony.

Support

Sometimes the alliances that independent midwives form surprised them: the supervisor of midwives who always seemed so out of touch before becomes their staunch supporter and their first port of call when experiencing a difficulty — a true 'guide, counsellor and friend'. Many GPs are very supportive of independent midwives, recognising the same feeling within them that made them choose general practice as a medical student. They will support, provide medical backup or will just be available on the other end of the telephone if ever the midwife needs to 'inform' a doctor of anything untoward.

There are however great disadvantages in independent practice. Not all independent midwives find a supportive supervisor, nor do they all find supportive GPs. Many feel extremely isolated and alone, sometimes frightened and unsure, and are aware of being seen as a menace and 'unsafe' by more orthodox practitioners.

The saddest aspect of the midwifery profession is that because it is a threatened group it tends to turn in upon itself, and the greatest delight of many midwives is criticising their colleagues in order to feel better about themselves. This is destructive to the profession as a whole, to the person who is being criticised and to the people who are doing the criticising, but at this stage in the profession's development, it may be inevitable. The great blessing for independent midwives is that they can always ring each other up at any time of the day or night and ask for help and advice and support, and as many of the midwives are very experienced, this can be very supportive.

The threat to the system

The fact that independent midwives are outside the system means that they can be seen as a threat to the local obstetricians, GPs and supervisors of midwives. Their practice may be different from the practice of in-hospital midwives because of their assumption of normality. The sort of women they attract may be more assertive than many others and thus may insist on certain practices when other women might be intimidated into compliance. This can make it difficult for those working in more orthodox situations to feel supportive.

- I well remember transferring a woman into the same hospital to which I had transferred another woman during the previous week. When I said to the registrar, 'Joan does not want continuous monitoring even though she is going to have syntocinon, but she will agree to our listening to the fetal heart regularly with our sonicaids', the registrar raised her eyebrows and said to me, 'Golly, Caroline, you do have difficult patients.' I was absolutely taken aback for a second because I have never perceived the women that we look after as 'difficult'. My response to the doctor was, 'No, they are not difficult, they are just challenging and interesting.' The doctor herself was an exceedingly kind, caring and compassionate doctor, but she had never been in a situation in which she was able to get to know people as well as I had. Most women she had looked after were too intimidated to do anything but comply, which is a difficulty about working with large numbers of women.

Moral dilemmas

With independent midwifery, there are enormous moral dilemmas. For instance, a woman may have a breech presentation and, despite advice to he contrary, decide to be booked for home delivery, the independent midwife having explained all the dangers surrounding a breech delivery generally and in particular a breech delivery at home. The woman may listen to the advice and then decide not to take the advice and to stay at home. The midwife, mindful of her role as 'mid-wife' — 'with woman' — supports the woman in her decision despite not agreeing with it. According to the Midwife's Code of Practice, the midwife informs the supervisor of midwives and continues with the care of the mother, but she may be disturbed by the reaction of the supervisor, who may imply that if she tried harder, she could 'persuade' the woman to go into hospital.

The independent midwife has a relationship with the woman in which 'bullying' has no place. Only true professional advice is given; sometimes it is accepted and sometimes it is rejected, but it is always the woman herself who decides. So how does the midwife feel if, after having gone through all the steps described, the worst nightmare of all occurs and the baby dies or perhaps even worse, is born asphyxiated and suffers a degree of brain damage? How does she feel now about supporting women against her own advice? Sometimes the weight of responsibility surrounding the work of an independent midwife is very, very heavy.

Supervision

Because of the great difference in philosophy between some independent midwives and their supervisors, many of whom have no experience of home birth or of independent practice, conflict can arise, and independent midwives appear to be very vulnerable to excessive 'supervision', 'investigation', 'suspension from practice' and referral to the professional conduct machinery. Consequently, they feel very much under threat and unable to trust or confide in their supervisors. The problem is exacerbated in London where each independent midwife is working in several health authorities and can at any one time have up to 100 different supervisors of midwives asking to see her equipment, records, drugs and books and criticising her practice, all in essence to protect the public's safety. But when the public that the midwife deals with is patently more than happy with the care received from the midwife, it seems extraordinary that so many independent midwives are being investigated by their supervisors. The whole system is in transition and is a source of discussion for the profession. Midwives are trying to work out better ways of being supervised, and supervisors of midwives are trying to work out better ways of supervising midwives' practice. In many areas it works very well, with supervisors enhancing the professional practice of midwives in their areas, being supportive and enabling the midwife to work in a professional way.

It is time that the role of the supervisor of midwives is looked into. It was a role that was inserted in the Midwives Act by medical practitioners to ensure that some supervision was kept over midwives, but it is interesting to note that no doctor has a supervisor of doctors who can intervene in his relationship with his professional body or in his relationship with his patient. Likewise, no dentist has a supervisor of dentists, who can pull him up on a point of clinical practice with which he does not agree. All clinical practice varies according to the perceived needs of that client at that time. In retrospect, we can all be perfect practitioners, but at the time, each midwife does as she thinks is best. Unless her decision is so gross and so extreme in its danger, she should not fear instant retribution but be given a chance to show that this was appropriate at that time for that woman, and because she has shown a consistent pattern of good midwifery practice, she should be safe from censure. At the moment the opposite is true. A midwife with an unblemished professional record can make one inadvertent slip and can instantly be suspended from practice and eventually struck off the register. All this is being debated within the profession. Injustice and harassment of a group hurts all members of that group, and for the sake of women, midwives need to feel strong and powerful.

The Importance of Childbirth

Childbirth reflects how a culture treats women. When women are immobilised and infantilised during labour, this is how society sees them, and the only people who are able to rescue women from this are strong midwives. When the midwifery profession tries to silence its more vociferous members — those who are less controllable and pliant because they work outside the system — the profession is working against women and, ultimately, against its own needs and professional growth. Eventually, this will be perceived by midwives; hopefully by then, it will not be too late. At the moment, the profession, which has always had a strong element of control from the medical profession, has managed to slough off the tentacles of the doctors, but is now in imminent danger of being taken over by the nursing profession — in the UK as it is throughout the world.

The reason why nurses are so attracted to encompassing the midwifery profession is because of the practitioner status of midwives, the limited prescribing rights, the statutory refresher courses, the living register and the history. Midwives are resisting the takeover, but sometimes those midwives who have found it easy to comply with the medicalisation of childbirth — who themselves have only ever practised in hospital and who have never had their eyes opened to what the role of the midwife truly is — cannot see the huge and unbridgeable gulf that there is between nursing and true midwifery. They genuinely see themselves as post-graduate nurses, to the detriment of the profession and to the huge detriment of women, who are in danger of being swamped by 'kindly nurses' masquerading as midwives. They explain everything that they are going to 'do to' the woman with great sweetness and empathy, they carry out all procedures for the woman's 'own good' and are 'really only concerned about your baby, dear'. But all the while, the woman lies there compliant and infantilised, control and power slipping away from her. Her grip on motherhood and being strong like a tigress for her child withers and disappears under the barrage of kindness and concern.

The independent midwife is also affected by her work; she is someone who chooses to work outside the system because she can no longer bear to practise as an obstetric nurse. However, she then has to justify her practice to doctors and sometimes other midwives who have no concept of 'normal' labour, whose principal thought is, 'what if something should go wrong?', who carry out tasks 'just in case something should go wrong' and who fill the atmosphere of the labour ward with fear, which affects everyone working within it, especially the mother who is very intuitive during labour. The independent midwife works from a different paradigm and from a different world view.

After having carried out just a few independent deliveries, the midwife finds her eyes being opened more and more. She can never go back. She can never 'unsee' what is happening to women. She can never turn the clock back on her perceptions, and she finds herself seeing more and more the strategies that are used on women to get them into hospital, mainly to provide employment for those who probably have little concept of what they are engaged in. She transfers women into hospital when necessary and then watches, angry and helpless, while a baby with an Apgar score of 9 is 'resuscitated' by an overenthusiastic paediatrician and goes into shock with a pneumothorax, the mother being brightly told, 'Well it's a good job you came into hospital isn't it? This baby needs a special care baby unit.' The midwife feels that she must go along with the lie.

The ethical dilemma to go along with this lie is extremely difficult because the baby did not actually need resuscitating and the pneumothorax is iatrogenic, but to confess this would put a great weight on the woman who will feel badly about the fact that she has transferred to hospital. It may harm the relationship between the mother and the midwife and may destroy the woman's trust in doctors and the midwifery profession.

The midwife needed to transfer the woman because the fetal heart sounded erratic with her pinards and sonicaid. Once she is able to monitor with an electronic fetal heart monitor, it is obvious that everything is fine, but having asked for help she is receiving it in plenty. Everyone is kind and welcoming. She is pleased to be there in many ways because she was getting tired and felt isolated, and the supervisor in this district is extremely critical. Now that she has transferred a woman, the supervisor will look upon her differently and will respect her more. But what is happening to this baby? Because there was meconium stained liquor, a paediatrician needed to be present at delivery — hence the resuscitation. The woman ends up lying on a hard bed, totally vulnerable and unable to move around and take charge, and the baby is being harmed. The midwife is alone with these feelings. She cannot share them with the woman. The woman, in her disappointment, needs to feel that it was absolutely necessary for the safety of her baby that she should go into hospital, have all these extra people at the delivery and for the baby to be intubated and then to have to go to a Special Care Baby Unit. She does not need to hear that the midwife was unsure and was actually covering her back. The hospital staff and the supervisor will not even understand what the midwife means should she voice this to them.

Conclusion

The independent midwife, at this time in our history, is taking on all the conflicts within our profession. She is the spearhead and the scapegoat; by persevering, the conflicts will eventually resolve, but in the meantime, life can be very hard for the independent practitioner.

And what about ethical issues? What am I doing writing this for a book for nurses? Why have I done it? I am flattered to be asked, my ego is being stroked — but that makes my action even less ethical. I am certainly not doing it for the money — I wish I were! But does that mean that my ethical values could be won over by financial reward? I have to come to the conclusion that it is inappropriate for me, a midwife, to write in a book specifically for nurses, because of the misunderstandings this can generate and because of the long struggle many of us have engaged in, pointing out that midwifery and nursing are entirely different and separate professions, with a few common meeting places but with very different philosophical and ethical roots. I should not have done this . . . but I did . . . to highlight the dilemma.

References

The Association of Radical Midwives (1986) *The Vision — Proposals for the Future of the Maternity Services.* Ormskirk: ARM.
Cumberlege, J (1994) Profile. *New Generation,* **13**(1): 46.

Department of Health (1993) *Changing Childbirth. Report of the Expert Maternity Group.* London: HMSO.
Health Committee, House of Commons (1992) *Maternity Services* (The Winterton Report). London: HMSO.
Micklethwaite, P, Beard, R and Shaw, K (1978) Expectations of a pregnant woman in relation to her treatment. *BMJ*, **2**: 188–91.
Oakley, A (1974–79) Transition to motherhood Project, Unpublished data. University of London, Bedford College.
Oakley, A (1984) *Women Confined.* Oxford: Martin Robertson.
Parents Magazine (1983) Birth in Britain. A *Parents* special report. A survey of 7,500 women's views. p. 92.
Parents Magazine (1986) Birth: 9000 mothers speak out. Birth Survey 1986 — results. p. 128.
Royal College of Midwives (1987) *The Role and Education of the Future Midwife in the United Kingdom.* London: RCM.
Royal College of Obstetricians and Gynaecologists (1982) *Report of the RCOG Working Party on Antenatal and Intrapartum Care.* London: RCOG.
UKCC (1991) *A Midwife's Code of Practice.* London: UKCC.

Index

abortion 43
abuse 54–5
  see also female circumcision
ACAS (Advisory, Conciliation and Arbitration Service) 16
Access to Health Records Act (1990) 44
accountability
  and *Scope of Professional Practice* (UKCC document) 25–6, 62
  and service commitment 75
Acts of Parliament
  Access to Health Records Act (1990) 44
  Children Act (1989) 7
  Data Protection Act (1984) 21
  Employment Protection (Consolidation) Act (1978) 16–17, 18
  Hospital Complaints Procedure Act (1985) 7
  Mental Health Act (1983) 6
  NHS and Community Care Act (1990) 4–5, 6, 21
  Nurses, Midwives and Health Visitors Act (1979) 10–11, 62
Advisory, Conciliation and Arbitration Service (ACAS) 16
advocacy 45–7
  anxiety in acting as advocate 54
  caution in undertaking 45
  and facilitators 54
Airedale NHS Trust v. *Bland* (1993) 10
alternative therapies 51–2
ARM (Association of Radical Midwives) 93
Arthur, Dr Leonard 45–6
assessment of patients 66
Association of Radical Midwives (ARM) 93

autonomy
  vs control 31–2
  and the professional 4, 77–9

behaviour
  common laws 2
  differing perspectives of 2–3
  education process 3
  rules of 2–3
  shaping of, in children 1–2
  see also control; professional behaviour
Bland, Tony 46–9
blood transfusion, refusal to accept 53–4
Blyth v. *Birmingham Waterworks Co. Ltd.* (1856) 8
Bolam v. *Friern Hospital Management Committee* (1957) 9
breast cancer, treatment options 50–1
Bull and Another v. *Devon AHA* (1989) 29

care
  care orientation being lost 37–8
  caring as a skill 64–5
  case law influence on 8–9
  changing setting of 25–7
  duty of, definition 8–9
  erosion of standards 76
  holistic 78
  increasing emphasis on community care 25, 26
  see also standards of practice
case law
  Airedale NHS Trust v.*Bland* (1993) 10
  Blyth v. *Birmingham Waterworks Co. Ltd.* (1856) 8
  Bolam v. *Friern Hospital Management Committee* (1957) 9

Index

Bull and Another v. *Devon AHA* (1989) 29
Donaghue v. *Stevenson* (1932) 8–9
  influence on patient care 9
  limited value for nursing profession 9–10
  and negligence 8–9
  procedures for development of 10
  Wilsher v. *Essex AHA* (1986–88) 26
childbirth
  with independent midwifery 101–3
  medicalisation of 101, 110
  midwife's perspective of 111–13
  a normal process 100–1. 102–3, 111
  see also under midwifery, independent practice
Children Act (1989) 7
choice 53–6
circumcision, female 57–8
Code for Nurses (ICN) 13
Code of Professional Conduct (UKCC)
  additional guidelines for standards 14
  and advocacy 45
  development of 61–2
  difficulties caused by some clauses 15–16
  and education 67
  group interpretations of 15
  for guidance and as a professional standard 13–14
  and industrial action 17
  links with the law 14–15
  and misconduct 30–1
  and nurses' concerns about standards 28–9
  and responsibility for caring 65
  and whistleblowing 39–40
codes of practice
  Advisory, Conciliation and Arbitration Service (ACAS) 16
  ICN *Code for Nurses* 13
  for managers? 40, 73
  Midwife's Code of Practice 88–9, 108
  for social workers? 74

  see also Code of Professional Conduct; standards of practice
commitment, of the professional 68–72
community care, increasing emphasis on 25, 26
companionship, caring 80–1
competence 66, 67, 68
  see also education; standards of practice
conflict of values
  and the apportionment of blame 56
  becoming more public 79
  efficiency *vs* nursing ethics 41
  managers *vs* nurses 40–2
  marketplace perspectives 52, 56–7
  nursing *vs* medical ethics 45, 47, 48–9, 50
  ostracism of questioners 39
  profession *vs* employers 4–5
  in the Tony Bland case 46–9
  treatment options for breast cancer 50–1
control
  vs autonomy 31–2
  consent to 31
  influence of 25–31
  social, methods of 1–3
  see also professional behaviour; social control

Data Protection Act (1984) 21
delegated legislation 10–11
Department of Health, guidelines 20–1
discipline
  and local employment rules 18
  following misconduct 29–31
  as sanction against unwanted behaviour 24
  and the UKCC 74
dismissal, as sanction against unwanted behaviour 24
Donaghue v. *Stevenson* (1932) 8–9
dying patient
  nursing *vs* medical ethics 48–9
  quality of life 46, 49
  role of the nurse 48

Index

education
 in developing behaviour patterns 3
 diploma level studies 67–8
 health care assistants 28
 more for needs of medical profession 64
 for new work areas 66, 67, 68, 69–70, 71–2
 nurses' responsibility for 25–6
 Post-registration Education and Practice (PREP) 11, 26, 68
 and the professional 67–8
 squeeze on training budgets 27
 and staff development 69–70
 students' perspectives of ethics 49–50
 see also Project 2000
employment
 codes and policies 16–17
 gagging clauses in contracts 19
 local rules, see employment rules, local
 union activity 17
Employment Protection (Consolidation) Act (1978) 16–17, 18
employment rules, local
 disciplinary 18
 and employee consultation 20
 enforcement of 19–20
 procedure for drawing up 18–19
 standards of performance 19–20
empowerment, in midwifery practice 87–8
English National Board (ENB), Higher Award 68
ethical principles
 factors affecting 42–3
 above the law? 42
 within market orientation? 42
ethical values
 blindness to, through familiarity 55
 difficult to explain 55
 see also conflict of values
ethnic issues 57
European Union (EU), influence on national law 12–13

facilitators, for senior staff 54
families, role in control of behaviour 3
female circumcision 57–8

guidelines for practice
 Department of Health 20–1
 NHS Management Executive 21
 and NHS Trusts 22
 professional bodies and unions 22–3
 Regional Health Authorities 21
 see also codes of practice; United Kingdom Central Council

health care assistants 28
honesty, see truth-telling
Hospital Complaints Procedure Act (1985) 7
humanity, service to, and the professional 74–7

ICN (International Council of Nurses), Code for Nurses 13
identification, professional 72–4
industrial action, see strikes
information, for patients 43–5
informed consent 43–4
 absence of 53–4
 definition 43
interchangeability, of nurses 65–6, 67, 71–2
International Council of Nurses (ICN), Code for Nurses 13

Joint Board of Clinical Nursing Studies (JBCNS) 68

labour, see childbirth
language problems 44
law
 civil 5
 classifications 5–6
 criminal 5
 delegated legislation 10–11
 influence of European Union 12–13
 and misconduct 29–31
 and social control 2–3

see also Acts of Parliament; case law; negligence; statute law
love, in caring relationships 80

management
  changes in 36
  code of conduct for? 40, 73
  danger of actions for negligence 28
  different from leadership 36–7
  role of 36–7
marketing environment 4–5, 6
  and standards of care 52, 56–7
medical records, patients' access to 44–5
Mental Health Act (1983) 6
midwifery
  and continuity of care and carer 92–4
  criticism within profession 106
  danger of takeover by nursing profession 110–11
  dealing with healthy women 85, 87
  independent, *see* midwifery, independent practice
  midwives as employees 87
  midwives *vs* obstetric nurses 111
  a separate profession? 84, 85, 110–11, 113
  team midwifery 93
midwifery, independent practice
  choice, mother's 88–9, 95, 100, 107–8
  diary notes, as shared record 97–8
  equipment, responsibility for 91, 105
  ethical principles 85–91
  financial considerations 89–91
  first consultation 96–7
  health advice 88
  immediate access to carer 102
  initial contact 95–6
  ongoing care 97–9
  postnatal 103–4
  procedures 87–8
  reasons for choosing independent midwife 91–4
  threat to local system 107
  type of service 101–3
  woman-based care 95–9

see also midwives, in independent practice
Midwife's Code of Practice 88–9, 108
midwives, in independent practice
  benefits to 104–6
  building up relationship 96–7
  disadvantages for 106–10
  independence of 105–6
  moral dilemmas 107–8, 112–13
  supervision of 108–10
  support for 106
  see also midwifery, independent practice
misconduct
  definition 30
  disciplinary action 29–31
  outcomes 29–31
  UKCC involvements 30
motherhood 99–101

National Boards 67–8
National Health Service, *see* NHS *entries*
negligence
  case law 8–9
  civil law 5
  definition 8
  elements of 8
  employers' liability 26
  inexperience no excuse for 26
  nurses' liability 26
  and staff levels 28
NHS and Community Care Act (1990) 4–5, 6, 21
NHS Management Executive (NHSME), guidelines 21
NHS Trusts
  encouraging good practice 22
  gagging clauses in contracts 19
  own pay levels 24
NHSME (NHS Management Executive), guidelines 21
Nurse Alert campaign 41–2
nurses
  changing skill mix 76
  extended practice of 78

Index

interchangeability of? 65–6, 67, 71–2
as 'Jack of all trades' 69
job satisfaction 70
lack of support for 54
numbers required 27–9
politicisation of 77
qualities of 80
see also professionals
Nurses, Midwives and Health Visitors Act (1979) 10–11, 62
Nurses Rules 10–11
nursing, a conveyor belt job? 38
nursing assessment 66
nursing ethics, students' perspectives of 49–50
nursing process 65

obstetric nurses *vs* midwives 111
obstetricians, private care from 95

patient assessment 66
patient information 43–5
Patient's Charter 50
Pink, Graham 40
Post-registration Education and Practice (Project) (PREP(P)) 11, 26, 68
principles, *see* ethical principles
professional behaviour
  case law affecting 8–10
  codes of conduct 13–16
  and delegated legislation 10–11
  employment codes and policies 16–20
  European Union influence 12–13
  guidelines for practice 20–3
  legal controls on 5–13
  local rules and policies 18–20
  nature of 3–5
  reporting unacceptable standards of care 15–16, 28–9, 31
  rewards 23–4
  sanctions 24–5
  statute law affecting 6–8
  union activity 17
  see also behaviour; control; discipline

professional bodies and unions, guidelines 22–3
professionals
  autonomy and 4, 77–9
  characteristics of 3–4
  commitment 68–72
  conflicting loyalties to profession and to employers 4–5
  definition 63
  education 67–8
  identification 72–4
  limitation of involvement 81
  right to criticise 39–40
  service to humanity 74–7
  vocation 63–7
  see also professional behaviour
Project 2000
  effect on nursing profession 64
  emphasis on community care 26
  introduction of 11
  and nursing ethics 42, 49–50

qualifications, relevance to work area 69–70
quality of life, the dying patient 46, 49

RCM (Royal College of Midwives) 72, 93
RCN, *see* Royal College of Nursing
records, patients' access to 44–5
Regional Health Authorities, guidelines 21
registration, of nurses 65–6, 74
reinforcement theory 23
religious orders 76–7
research findings, demands for 37
resources, scarcity of 28–9
responsibility 75
rewards
  extrinsic 23–4
  intrinsic 23
  to shape behaviour 23
right to know 43–5
Royal College of Midwives (RCM) 72, 93
Royal College of Nursing (RCN)

educational programmes 72
ethical issues 72–3
and strike action 75
and whistleblowing 39–40

sanctions 24–5
Scope of Professional Practice (UKCC document)
  and accountability 25–6, 62
  extended practice of nurses 78
  and updating of knowledge and competence 67
  service to humanity, and the professional 74–7
shop stewards 17
social control, *see* control
social workers, code of conduct for? 74
staff development 69–70
standards of practice and performance
  in constantly changing environment 36
  erosion of 76
  local policies 19
  measurement of 41
  monitoring and facilitating 41
  nurses' attitudes to 36
  reporting concerns about 15–16, 28–9, 31
  and the UKCC 22, 40
  UKCC additional guidelines 14
  uniformity of care and treatment 38–9
  see also codes of practice
statute law
  difficulties of interpretation 7
  influencing 7–8
  procedures 8
  see also Acts of Parliament
strikes
  and codes of conduct 17
  RCN attitude to 75
  in the USA 75–6, 77
support for nurses, lack of 54–5

team midwifery 93
trade unions 17
  guidelines 22–3
training, *see* education
truth-telling, in midwifery practice 85–7

UKCC, *see* United Kingdom Central Council for Nursing, Midwifery and Health Visiting
unions, *see* trade unions
United Kingdom Central Council for Nursing, Midwifery and Health Visiting (UKCC)
  Council membership 62
  and delegated legislation 10–11
  disciplinary provisions 74
  guidelines on nursing standards 14, 22
  Midwife's Code of Practice 88–9, 108
  and misconduct 30
  Nurses Rules 10–11
  objectives 62
  and registration 74
  representative of nursing profession 62–3
  and standards of care 40
  see also Code of Professional Conduct; Post-registration Education and Practice; Scope of Professional Practice
United States of America (USA), nurses' strikes 75–6, 77

values, *see* ethical values
vocation, and the professional 63–7
  definition 74
  service to humanity 74–7
voluntary organisations 76–7

whistleblowing 39–40
Whitley Council 24, 29
Wilsher v. *Essex AHA* (1986–88) 26